Trazodone

Modern Problems of Pharmacopsychiatry

Vol. 9

S. Karger · Basel · München · Paris · London · New York · Sydney

Proceedings of the First International Symposium, Montreal, Que., October 1973

Trazodone

Volume Editors:
TH. A. BAN, Montreal, Que.
B. SILVESTRINI, Rome

With 86 figures and 83 tables, 1974

S. Karger · Basel · München · Paris · London · New York · Sydney

Modern Problems of Pharmacopsychiatry

Vol. 1: Clinical Psychopharmacology
X+284 p., 26 fig., 27 tab., 1968. ISBN 3-8055-0526-4
Vol. 2: The Thioxanthenes
X+118 p., 27 fig., 12 tab., 1969. ISBN 3-8055-0527-2
Vol. 3: Depression: Its Diagnosis and Treatment. Lithium: The History of its Use in Psychiatry
XIII+92 p., 14 tab., 1969. ISBN 3-8055-0528-0
Vol. 4: Epilepsy
VIII+340 p., 40 fig., 40 tab., 1970. ISBN 3-8055-0529-9
Vol. 5: The Neuroleptics
X+190 p., 38 fig., 9 tab., 1970. ISBN 3-8055-0530-2
Vol. 6: The Role of Drugs in Community Psychiatry
VI+128 p., 3 fig., 3 tab., 1971. ISBN 3-8055-1200-7
Vol. 7: Psychological Measurements in Psychopharmacology
VI+267 p., 25 fig., 54 tab., 1974. ISBN 3-8055-1630-4
Vol. 8: Psychotropic Drugs and the Human EEG
ca. 300 p., ca. 88 fig., ca. 19 tab., 1974. ISBN 3-8055-1419-0

S. Karger · Basel · München · Paris · London · New York · Sydney
Arnold-Böcklin-Strasse 25, CH-4011 Basel (Switzerland)

Printed in Switzerland by Buchdruckerei Berner Zeitung AG, 3550 Langnau
Blocks: Steiner & Co., Basel
ISBN 3-8055-1718-1

Table of Contents

First Clinical Session

Second Clinical Session

Free Communications Session

Third Clinical Session

Introduction

Whenever a new therapeutic substance is introduced to the scientific community numerous and complex problems, often unforeseen, seem to arise suddenly. These are problems not solely connected with therapeutic specificity, but of such a broad nature as to implicate the entire field of our basic knowledge.

These considerations are confirmed in this book, since throughout it, biochemical, pharmacological and clinical concepts are brought to a scrutiny which in the end raises more questions than provides answers. This book is, in fact, the result of a gathering of scientists and clinicians from many parts of the world, convened in Montreal to report findings and discuss results of a new psychoactive drug: trazodone.

Of these problems, some deserve a particular attention. Which criteria, for example, shall apply when we are called upon to determine whether a new substance deserves that huge investment both in terms of human efforts as well as economics necessary to transform a substance from a laboratory curiosity into a therapeutic entity?

Criteria which were valid in the past no longer apply. To an era of full confidence, which through dramatic discoveries has created the premises of present day medicine, a more cautious approach has followed with emphasis on toxicological problems. Now we are going through an era which I would classify as 'ecological' even with regard to medicinal pharmacy. Not only researchers but also politicians and laymen have recognized that the use of drugs may alter delicate biological balances; and not only in humans, but also in our environment. As a consequence, we have become much more strict in defining the features of drugs suitable for development. And while a satisfactory therapeutic response is still a basic requirement, it is no longer considered sufficient by itself. Now we are looking for new mechanisms, new modes of action; or, alternatively if not concomitantly, for drugs which are useful in fields where nothing effective is available; or where the therapeutic measures at our disposal are too risky in terms of possible toxicity. The Montreal meeting on trazodone has revealed this mood in the international scientific community; and trazodone itself, as a new drug, appears particularly appropriate as a focal point for these considerations. Here we have, in fact, a substance with unusual pharmacological features, as well as uncommon therapeutic properties.

The meeting on trazodone was a good opportunity for discussing another problem of general interest, namly the methodology of psychopharmacological research. It is generally recognized that the discovery of modern psychotropic drugs is closely connected, as far as experimental research is concerned, to the development of the so-called 'drug-shaped' methodology.

Since basic knowlege of mental mechanisms is unsatisfactory, pharmacologists have used known drugs already established in human use to formalize their experimental models and interpret the results.

However, we are no longer solely interested in derivatives of known chemical series which provide quantitative and not qualitative improvements. We are looking for new mechanisms or mode of action, or for efficacy in otherwise incurable diseases.

While on the medical level there is an ever-increasing demand for entirely 'new' psychoactive drugs, the 'drug-shaped' research is only capable of recognizing the potential value of substances which present substantial similarities with already known drugs.

Experience gained with trazodone demonstrates that the basic knowledge presently available is adequate for a different approach to research.

To evidence this point let me record the conclusive findings of animal pharmacology which preceded the clinical trials on trazodone. Following the conventional 'drug-shaped' approach this drug did not reveal any significant similarities with antidepressive drugs, whereas some data could suggest its classification among neuroleptics. Nevertheless, the antidepressive activity of trazodone, which has been subsequently recognized in humans, was foreseen on the basis of an original interpretation of animal findings and expressed in this way: 'theoretical speculations would suggest a preferential use of AF 1161 in depressive disorders'. The rationale for such an interpretation has already been illustrated in the first pharmacological paper published on this drug [Silvestrini *et al.*, 1968] and in occasion of the Round Table Discussion on Trazodone held in Amsterdam last June [Silvestrini and Lisciani, 1973].

Unfortunately, even in psychopharmacology conventional interpretations enjoy, as a rule, a much greater acceptance than new approaches, as demonstrated by the fact that in some literature on trazodone the following introductory statement is reported: 'animal data suggested a neuroleptic activity of trazodone'.

I think that we should fight against this mental attitude. In fact, medical research should look to the future without being conditioned by conventional schemes.

I would like to conclude with a personal touch. In 1968, preliminary clinical data on trazodone were presented at a meeting of the World Psychiatric Association. At that time Thomas Ban was present and already at that early stage of development foresaw the potentialities of this drug. The studies which followed confirmed these previsions. On this occasion I want to thank Thomas Ban for his fundamental contributions to the understanding of this drug.

B. Silvestrini

Pharmacology Session

Chairman: C. RADUCO-THOMAS

Trazodone. Mod. Probl. Pharmacopsychiat., vol. 9, pp. 4–10,
ed. Th. A. Ban, Montreal, Que., and B. Silvestrini, Rome (Karger, Basel 1974)

Pharmacological Features of Trazodone

V. G. LONGO and A. SCOTTI DE CAROLIS
Istituto Superiore di Sanità, Roma

The advent of what is called the chemotherapy of mental diseases goes back to the years 1952–1953, when chlorpromazine was introduced in the treatment of various psychiatric conditions, followed by reserpine, which had similar applications, and by meprobamate for the relief of anxiety. The first observations dealing with their usefulness in psychiatric patients originated in the clinic.

The outburst of research which followed the reports of the positive therapeutic effects of the new drugs was characterized by a close cooperation between pharmacologists and clinicians; the advent of this collaboration constitutes the birth of neuropsychopharmacology as a new discipline.

Following a period of intense activity, which lasted some ten years, a phase of evaluation ensued. Countless congresses, symposia and round table conferences followed one another with the purpose of classifying the various actions of drugs, comparing their effects on man with the experimental animal data; new interdisciplinary organizations and publications contributed to the dissemination of pertinent data. The task of classsifying and characterizing the new pharmaceuticals proved arduous. This difficulty is reflected by numerous attempts at the 'taxonomy' of these products.

By 1967, neuropsychopharmacology had grown into a major scientific discipline. I mention this date because in that year the American College of Neuropsychopharmacology organized in Puerto Rico a meeting celebrating the 10th anniversary of its foundation. During this meeting many facets of this discipline, both facts and hypotheses, were discussed by an international scientific group. The proceedings were then published in a monstrous volume of 1,500 pages, which is still considered as the Bible of this field [EFRON *et al.*, 1968].

Today, like all established sciences, neuropsychopharmacology is caracterized by its own type of research, apparatus and special procedures.

In the laboratory, these procedures were designed to parallel as closely as possible pathological states in man. However, as we all well know, this model-relationship is seldom, if ever, obtained. For this reason, laboratory methods were derived from the results observed in man in an empirical way, which can be schematized as follows: if different classes of drugs have qualitatively different effects in humans, attempts are made to demonstrate qualitatively different effects of these drugs in animals, regardless of the tests used to show such differences. After the effects of standard drug classes are established in animal tests, new compounds are examined by these procedures, and their effects compared with the standard drugs.

Considering that so little is known about the fundamental causes of the mental diseases, this approach is considered the only safe one. Unfortunately, such a selection procedure markedly reduces the likelihood of discovering something significantly novel or different. In other words, our present methods are inadequate for the exploration of new problems.

The table summarizes the principal methods used in the laboratory for screening the three major classes of drugs used in the chemotherapy of mental diseases; the antipsychotics, the antidepressants and the antianxiety agents (table I).

The 50 or so drugs which are presently employed in psychiatry arrived at the point of human trials because of laboratory screening made with the aforementioned techniques. In these last years, however, a number of drugs have appeared which did not fit any classical schema. There are two principal mechanisms through which this happened. The first is certainly due to the initiative of some enlightened researchers whose interest did not falter in spite of the fact that laboratory tests were unable to pigeonhole the drug into the existing schemes.

The second mechanism has taken advantage of the progress in the investigations on the biochemical mechanism of mental diseases, utilizing molecules which, although not necessarily fitting any preordained outline, demonstrated nevertheless antagonism or interference with neurotransmission mechanisms thought to be implicated in mental diseases.

The results thus obtained, although not particularly glamorous, allow us to affirm that there are some antipsychotics which do not induce sedation or catalepsy in animals; that there are some antidepressants which do not antagonize the effects of reserpine in rats; that there are some antianxiety agents without any muscle-relaxing or taming effects in animals.

A drug which seems to fall into the category of compounds not easily placed into any preordained scheme is trazodone; and I would like now to

Table I.
Tests used in the laboratory for the evaluation of potential psychotropic drugs

Profile of activity for antipsychotics
Sedative effects (diminution of spontaneous motility or curiosity, inhibition of aggressive behavior, enhancement of other CNS depressants)
Cataleptic effects
Disruption of conditioned avoidance responses
Antagonistic effects (block of stereotype behavior due to amphetamine, L-dopa or apomorphine; protection from group toxicity due to amphetamine; antiemetic effects)
Neurovegetative effects (α-adrenolytic action)
Profile of activity for antidepressants
Antagonism of reserpine or tetrabenazine sedation
Anticataleptic action
Central anticholinergic effects
L-Dopa potentiation
Profile of activity for antianxiety agents
Muscle-relaxing effect (decerebrate rigidity, polysynaptic reflexes)
Anticonvulsant action
Taming of spontaneous and elicited vicious behavior
Attenuation of various types of conflict behavior

discuss the pharmacological characteristics of trazodone, in the light of published work and of results obtained in our laboratory.

Trazodone is inactive in standard tests for antidepressant agents, i. e., reserpine antagonism or L-dopa potentiation; it is not a MAO inhibitor; it differs from the antianxiety agents because it lacks anticonvulsant effects and its muscle-relaxing action is very weak, even though in our laboratory [LOIZZO and MASSOTTI, 1973] trazodone was found to have a certain taming action on septal rats (fig. 1).

Assessment of the antipsychotic activity of trazodone in the laboratory yielded the following results: the drug inhibits an avoidance-conditioned response at doses which do not influence the unconditioned reaction, and protects mice from amphetamine group toxicity [SILVESTRINI *et al.*, 1968]. It lacks, however, significant cataleptogenic properties, has weak hypothermic activity and does not inhibit the stereotyped behavior due to amphetamine or apomorphine. In regard to peripheral effects, trazodone has a spectrum of activity different from other neuroleptics: it is very effective against serotonin, mildly active on epinephrine and norepinephrine and practically inactive against L-dopa, histamine and acetylcholine.

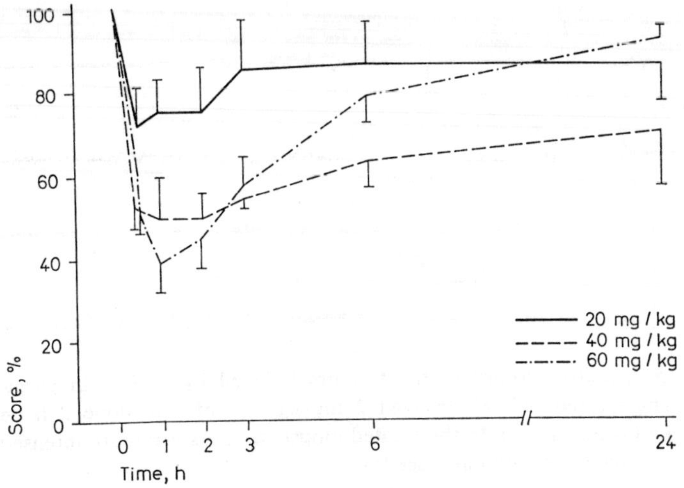

Fig. 1. Effect of trazodone on septal hyperirritability in rats. Ordinate: irritability scores expressed as percent on the control score before drug. Abscissa: time in hours (injection at time 0). Each curve represents the mean ± SE of at least three animals treated with the indicated dose of the drug [from LOIZZO and MASSOTTI, 1973].

Some additional data relevant to possible mechanism of action of the drug should be mentioned. One of its effects is the attenuation of the reaction of discomfort and pain, as assessed by the phenylquinone writhing test or by the grooming test [SILVESTRINI and QUADRI, 1970; YAMATSU *et al.*, 1972]. It seems, in fact, that trazodone acts with a peculiar selectivity in conditions characterized by the activation of mechanisms of emotional integration of unpleasant experiences. These data have suggested some clinical applications of trazodone. Other data, which Dr. YAMATSU will present in more detail in this session, deal with the suppression of paradoxical sleep in the rat, after doses of 10 and 40 mg/kg p. o. This effect was accompanied by a decrease of 5HIAA level in whole brain.

This interference with the central serotoninergic system may be related to some data obtained in our laboratory in the course of studies on the influence of trazodone on the behavioral effects of L-dopa and 5-HTP in mice.

One of the pharmacological tests used in the laboratory for the evaluation of antidepressant drugs is the L-dopa potentiation in mice [EVERETT, 1967]. Potentiation obtained with tricyclic drugs has been attributed to an inhibition of the norepinephrine uptake mechanisms at the nerve terminals;

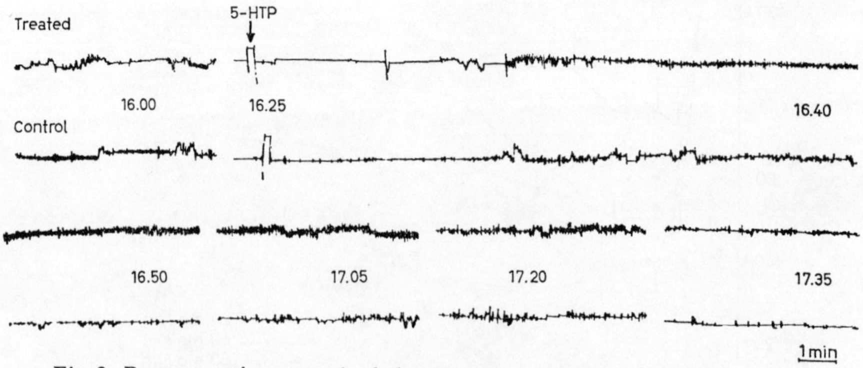

Fig. 2. Representative record of the tremors induced by 5-HTP in pargyline-treated mice. The treated animal received 2 mg/kg i. p. of trazodone 2 h before 5-HTP 75 mg/kg (at the arrow). In the treated mouse, tremors are more intense than in the control. For details of technique, see text.

this causes a high concentration of the mediator at the central synaptic site, with resulting greater pharmacological effects. There is still much controversy on the biochemical etiology of the affective disorders, and both catecholamines and indoleamines have been involved. For instance, results of Carlsson *et al.* [1968] in the rat indicate that imipramine blocks *in vivo* the uptake mechanisms in central serotoninergic synapses. Clinical data also suggest both type of transmitters may be involved: patients suffering from a depressive illness improve following large doses of tryptophan combined with a MAO inhibitor [Coppen, 1968].

In our investigations, trazodone was found to be ineffective on the L-dopa potentiation test. However, when tried on the behavioral effects of 5-HTP, it proved to be very active. In mice pretreated with a MAO-inhibitor, 5-HTP induces head twitchings and whole-body tremors, ensuing 5–10 min after i. p. injection, and lasting for about one hour. When mice receive in advance trazodone, in doses as low as 2 mg/kg i. p., the tremors induced by 5-HTP arise earlier, are more intense, and last longer than in control animals (fig. 2). Moreover, when the tremors and the incoordinated activity fade away, a noticeable increase in the spontaneous activity and exploration appears, which lasts for 2 h (fig. 3).

The patterns of 5-HTP potentiation observed with trazodone strongly resemble that obtained in mice treated with an intracerebral injection of 5,6-dihydroxytryptamine (5,6-DHT) [Longo *et al.,* 1973]. In this case, 5-HTP enhancement was attributed to an impaired uptake of the mediator due to the destruction of nerve terminals caused by 5,6-DHT.

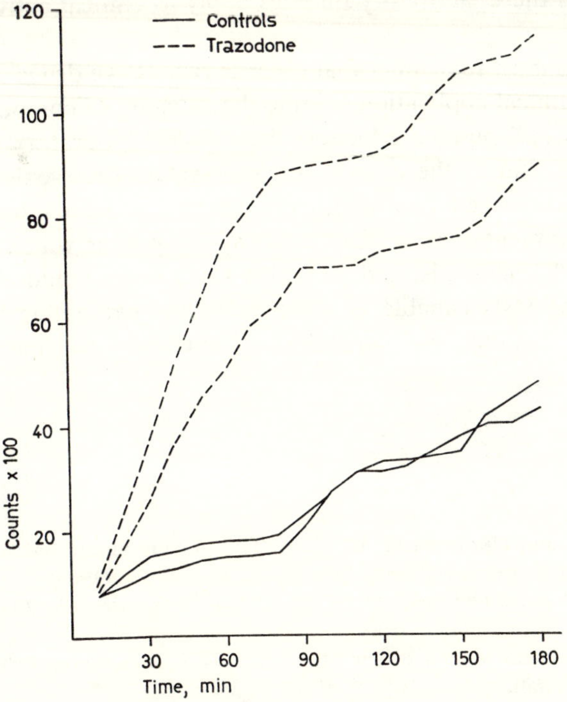

Fig. 3. Effect of 5-HTP on spontaneous activity of pargyline-treated mice. Cumulative records of four groups of 5 mice each (Animex apparatus); 5-HTP (75 mg/kg) injected at time 0. The broken lines show the scores obtained in animals treated with 2 mg/kg of trazodone 2 h before 5-HTP. The continuous lines show the response of control mice. Ordinate: printouts of Animex counter; abscissa: time in minutes.

Another drug which induces 5-HTP potentiation is the thyrotropin releasing hormone (TRH) [Huidobro-Toro *et al.*, 1973], for which an antidepressant effect in man has been reported recently. Our results offer some leads which may be relevant to the identification of the mechanism of action, or of one of the mechanisms of action of trazodone; namely an inhibition of the uptake of the mediator at the central serotoninergic terminals. I am sure that further investigations on the levels and on the turnover of brain amines could contribute to the clarification of these effects. Perhaps Dr. Garattini could enlighten us on this point.

I hope this talk has presented fairly the efforts of pharmacologists to isolate and identify the various activities of trazodone. To what extent and in which relationships these laboratory findings apply to clinical activity is hard to say.

In this context we must remember that other psychoactive drugs which have recently found clinical application fall into the category of compounds which do not possess indisputable effects in the classical laboratory tests. Perhaps the reason is that in the central nervous system there exists, in addition to the acknowledged operating mechanisms on which usually impinges all our experimentation, a silent majority of systems which contribute to the central homeostasis, and on which some drugs could act. It is our task to develop tests capable of discovering and evaluating these systems, in order to enhance our capability of screening possible new psychopharmaca.

References

CARLSSON, A.; FUXE, K., and UNGERSTEDT, U.: The effect of imipramine on central 5-hydroxytryptamine neurons. J. Pharm. Pharmacol. *20:* 150–151 (1968).

COPPEN, A. J.: Depressed states and indolealkylamines. Adv. Pharmacol. *6B:* 283–291 (1968).

EFRON, D. H.: Psychopharmacology: a review of progress (US Government Printing Office, Washington 1968).

EVERETT, G. M.: in GARATTINI and DUKES Antidepressant drugs, pp. 166–167 (Excerpta Medica Foundation, Amsterdam 1967).

HUIDOBRO-TORO, J. P.; SCOTTI DE CAROLIS, A., and LONGO, V. G.: Action of two hypothalamic factors (TRH, MIF) and of angiotensin II on the behavioral effects of L-dopa and 5-HTP in mice. Pharmacol. Biochem. Behav. *2:* 86–89 (1974).

LOIZZO, A. and MASSOTTI, M.: Taming effects of nonnarcotic analgesics on the septal syndrome in rats. Pharm. Biochem. Behav. *1:* 367–370 (1973).

LONGO, V. G.; SCOTTI DE CAROLIS, A.; LIUZZI, A., and MASSOTTI, M.: A study on the central effects of 5,6-DHT. In COSTA and SANDLER Advances in Biochemical Psychopharmacology, vol. 10 and 11, Serotonin – New Vistas (Raven Press, New York 1974).

SILVESTRINI, B.; CIOLI, V.; BURBERI, S., and CATANESE, B.: Pharmacological properties of AF 1161, a new psychotropic drug. Int. J. Neuropharmacol. *7:* 587–599 (1968).

SILVESTRINI, B. and QUADRI, E.: Investigations on the specificity of the so-called analgesic activity of non-narcotic drugs. Eur. J. Pharmacol. *12:* 231–235 (1970).

YAMATSU, K.; KANEKO, T.; YAMANISHI, Y.; KITAHARA, A., and OHTAKE, S.: A Possible Mechanism of Central Action of Trazodone in Rats. Mod. Probl. Pharmacopsych., vol. 9, pp. 11–17 (Karger, Basel 1974).

Author's address: Prof. V. G. LONGO, Istituto Superiore di Sanità, *I-00161 Roma* (Italy)

Trazodone. Mod. Probl. Pharmacopsychiat., vol. 9, pp. 11–17,
ed. Th. A. Ban, Montreal, Que., and B. Silvestrini, Rome (Karger, Basel 1974)

A Possible Mechanism of Central Action of Trazodone in Rats

K. Yamatsu, T. Kaneko, Y. Yamanishi, A. Kitahara and S. Ohtake

Department of Pharmacology, Section of Experimental Therapeutics Research, Research and Development Division, Eisai Co. Ltd., Tokyo

Introduction

It has been shown by Silvestrini *et al.* [1968] and Silvestrini and Quadri [1970] that trazodone has an unusual spectrum of pharmacological activity and cannot easily be classified among the classes of already known psychotropic drugs.

Furthermore, in our investigations [Yamatsu *et al.*, 1972], as summarized in figure 1, the following pharmacological features were recognized: trazodone specifically suppresses the response (writhing or grooming behaviour) to painful or unpleasant stimuli at doses (less than 10 mg/kg p. o.) which did not change motor activity in mice. In contrast, this compound does not possess anticonvulsant properties, anti-tremorine activity, anti-reserpine activity or cataleptogenic properties even at a dose of 160 mg/kg.

On the other hand, it has been shown that trazodone has potent anti-serotonin activities, i. e. antagonisms against the serotonin bronchial constriction *in vivo* [Silvestrini *et al.*, 1968] and against the contraction of isolated rat stomach produced by serotonin [Kaneko *et al.*, 1972]. These findings are interesting especially in regard to the mechanism of central actions of trazodone.

This study was designed to investigate the effects of trazodone on the serotonergic system in the brain and the mechanisms possibly involved in its central actions in rats.

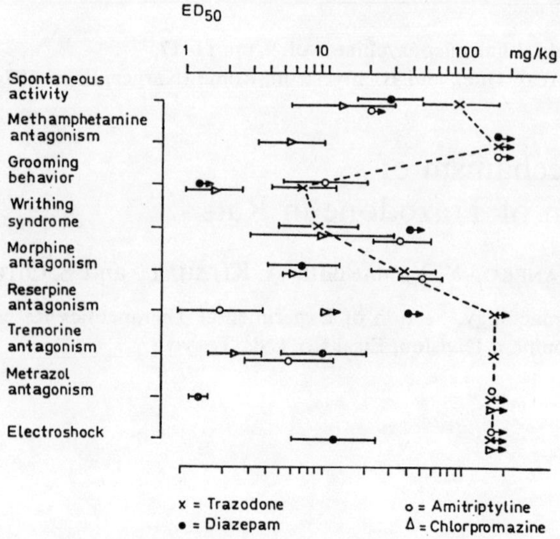

Fig. 1. Comparison of the pharmacological profile of trazodone with that of diazepam, amitriptyline or chlorpromazine in mice. ED_{50} value obtained 50–70 min after oral administration of drugs. Horizontal bar, 95% confidence limits. Arrow, either dose-response slope too shallow to be calculated for confidence limits or little effect at a maximal dose level.

Experimental

1. Effect on the Sleep-Wakefulness Cycle in Rats

The effect of trazodone on the sleep-wakefulness cycle during daytime was compared with that of imipramine, diazepam or chlorpromazine in rats.

Male Wistar rats bearing chronically implanted electrodes were used for electro-encephalographic and myographic recordings.

Continuous recordings were conducted during 7 or 10 h after oral administration of drugs or vehicle (saline or 5% arabic gum). Control recordings were done on the day prior to treatment and on the treatment day (2nd day), 2–3 h before the administration of drugs.

All results of recordings were expressed as the means of three animals per dose, with the exception of control recordings which included 12 measurements.

Analysis of data was done by dividing the tracing into blocks of 10 sec which corresponded to an integral period of EEG, and as shown in figure 2 each block of 10 sec was defined as slow wave sleep, paradoxical sleep, or wakefulness on the basis of the criteria described by JACOBS and MCGINTY [1971].

In the controls, 85.2% of the recordings taken during a 10-hour period resulted in sleeping time, whereas 14.8% was paradoxical sleep (table I).

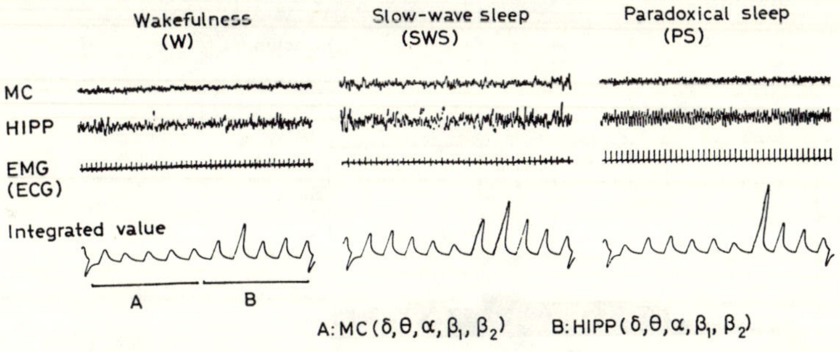

Fig. 2. Sleep-wakefulness parameters in rats. MC, motor cortex; HIPP, hippocampus; integrated value, integrated values for 10 sec of five frequency bands of the cortical and hippocampal EEG.

Table I. Summary of the effects of trazodone on sleep-wakefulness cycle in rats

	Control vehicle	Trazodone, mg/kg 2.5[1]	10[1]	40	160
Percent time of each phase					
W/RT	25.4	24.9	30.7	30.8	59.4
SWS/RT	59.8	59.1	60.8	62.7	40.6
PS/RT	14.8	15.9	8.5	6.5	0
Latency to onset of PS hours and min	41 m	1 h 01 m	1 h 19 m	5 h 02 m	10 h
Duration of PS, min	2.3	2.9	2.0	2.5	–
Numbers of PS/h	3.9	3.1	2.7	1.6	–
Duration of SWS, min					
Sw	3.7	3.3	4.2	5.9	7.8
Sp	5.3	6.9	7.3	7.0	–

Three rats per dose were orally administered an increasing dose of trazodone. Control, n = 12.
W, wakefulness; SWS, slow wave sleep; PS, paradoxical sleep; Sw, SWS followed by W. Sp, SWS followed by PS; RT, recording time of 10 h.
1 RT of 7 h.

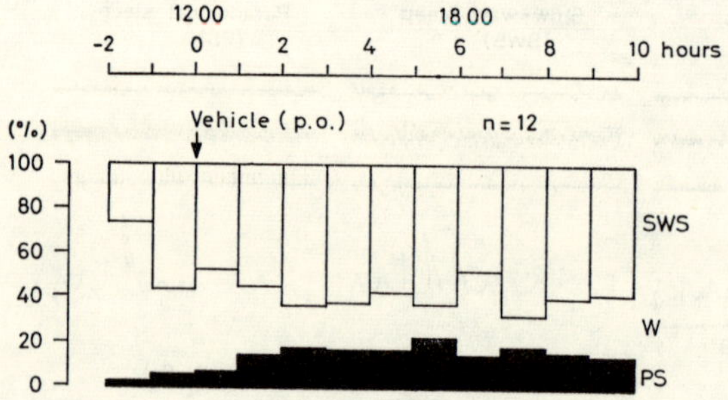

Percent time of each phase	W/RT	25.4
	SWS/RT	59.8
	PS/RT	14.8
Latency to onset of PS		41 min
Duration of PS		2.3 min
Numbers of PS/h		3.9
Duration of SWS	SW	3.7 min
	SP	5.3 min

W = Wakefulness
SWS = Slow wave sleep
PS = Paradoxical sleep
SW = SWS followed by W
SP = SWS followed by PS
RT = Recording time of 10 h

Fig. 3. Hourly pattern of slow wave sleep, paradoxical sleep and wakefulness in control recordings.

Trazodone at a dose of 10 mg/kg decreased paradoxical sleep during 7 h following administration; no effect was observed at a dose of 2.5 mg/kg.

At the dose of 40 mg/kg trazodone delayed the onset of the first phase of paradoxical sleep and caused a noticeable and selective suppression of paradoxical sleep for about 7 h; no significant change of slow wave sleep was observed (fig. 3).

As shown in figure 3 and table I, the highest dose (160 mg/kg) reduced slow wave sleep, accompanied by a decrease in amplitude of the hippocampal EEG. At the same time no change of excitable gross behaviour was noticed, whereas remarkable sedation (lasting for more than 10 h) was evident. All animals at the highest dose failed to have episodes of paradoxical sleep during the entire recording period.

When compared with trazodone, diazepam exerted no effect on the sleep-wakefulness cycle with doses (40 mg/kg) large enough to cause marked muscle relaxation; background activities of cortical and hippocampal tracings were altered. Moreover, chlorpromazine at a dose of 10 mg/kg produced a change characterized by a predominant theta rhythm of hippocampal EEG and suppressed the onset of typical paradoxical sleep for more than 7 h.

Imipramine at 10 and 40 mg/kg (but not at 2.5 mg/kg) produced marked decrease or loss of paradoxical sleep with slight decrease of slow wave sleep during 7 h following dosing.

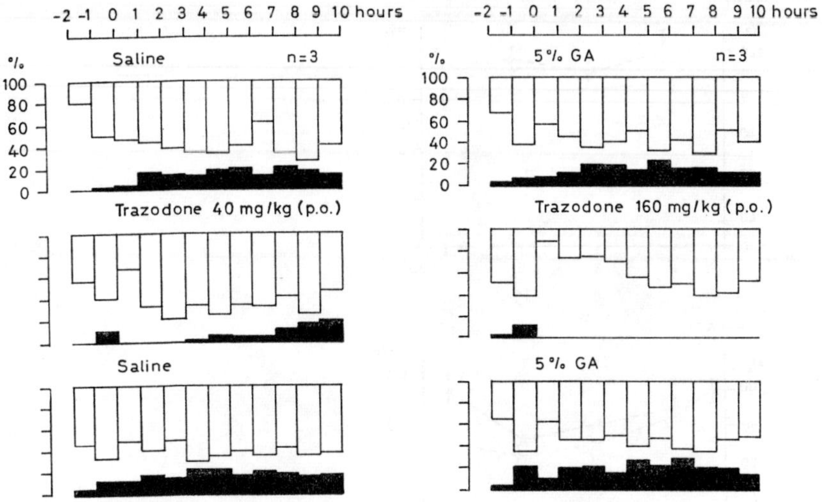

Fig. 4. Time courses of effects of 40 and 160 mg/kg of trazodone on the daytime sleep-wakefulness cycle in rats. Trazodone was given orally on the 2nd day of the experiments. The results are the means of three rats per dose. White columns, slow-wave sleep; black columns, paradoxical sleep; other areas, wakefulness. 5% GA, 5% gummi arabic solution. A represents the 1st day of the experiment, B the 2nd day, C the 3rd day.

Imipramine caused selective suppression of paradoxical sleep in a dose which produced anti-reserpine activity in rats or mice [Khazan and Brown, 1970; Yamatsu and Kaneko, 1973].

Thus, the effect of trazodone on the sleep-wakefulness cycle in rats appears to be noticeably different from that of diazepam or chlorpromazine and may be comparable to that of imipramine. However, in contrast to imipramine, trazodone had no anti-reserpine activity at a dose which selectively suppressed paradoxical sleep. Therefore, other mechanisms than that of imipramine should be considered for the paradoxical sleep suppressing effect of trazodone in rats.

2. *Effects on the Levels of Monoamines in the Rat Brain*

Experiments were performed to investigate whether trazodone produces neurochemical changes at doses (40 and 160 mg/kg) which affect sleep-wakefulness cycle.

Male Wistar rats weighing 250–300 g were used. Four rats in each group were given trazodone p. o. or saline and sacrificed after 1, 3, 5 and 7 h.

The concentrations of noradrenaline (NA), dopamine (DA), 5-hydroxytryptamine (5-HT) and 5-hydroxyindolacetic acid (5-HIAA) in the whole brain were estimated spectrofluorometrically with the same tissue sample by the methods of Chang [1964] and Miller *et al.* [1970].

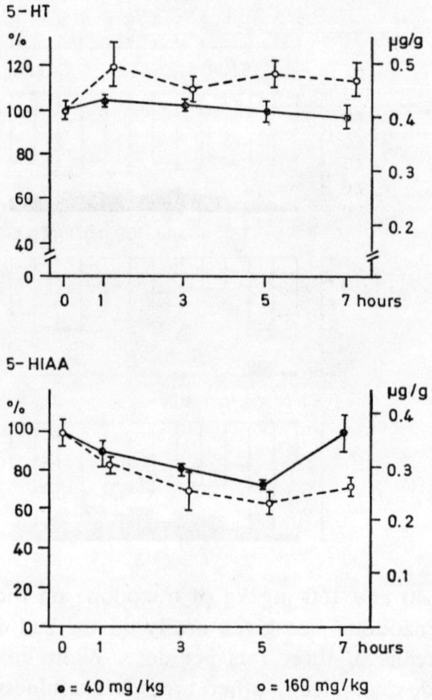

Fig. 5. Effects of trazodone on the levels of 5-hydroxytryptamine (5-HT) and 5-hydroxyindolacetic acid (5-HIAA) in the whole brain of rats. Four rats in each group were administered orally with trazodone 40 mg/kg, 160 mg/kg or vehicle and then killed after 0, 1, 3, 5 and 7 h. All results are expressed as mean ±SEM (n = 4).

At doses of 40 and 160 mg/kg trazodone produced no significant effect on the levels of NA and DA in the whole brain. On the other hand, at the dose level of 160 mg/kg, there was small but definite increase in the level of 5-HT in the brain which reached a maximum at 1 h and lasted for more than 7 h.

In addition to the increase of brain 5-HT, trazodone produced a noticeable decrease in the level of 5-HIAA in the rat brain at doses of 40 and 160 mg/kg, as shown in figure 4. Trazodone at 40 mg/kg decreased the 5-HIAA level to about 80% of control level 3–5 h following administration; the 5-HIAA level was recovered to control levels 7 h after dosing. Decrease in brain 5-HIAA level following dosing of 160 mg/kg trazodone was greater in degree than with 40 mg/kg and lasted longer.

Effects of trazodone on the levels of 5-HT and 5-HIAA in the rat brain appeared to be dose-dependent.

At a dose of 40 mg/kg, which selectively suppressed paradoxical sleep, trazodone caused a decrease in the 5-HIAA level in the whole rat brain.

Furthermore, changes in the brain level of 5-HIAA after dosing of trazodone at doses of 40 and 160 mg/kg and suppression of paradoxical sleep displayed almost similar time patterns.

Conclusions

On the basis of the findings obtained, it is suggested that the central actions of trazodone in rats is primarily attributable to its effect on the serotonergic system rather than on the catecholaminergic system in the brain.

These possible mechanisms of central action of trazodone may provide a tentative basis for the interpretation of clinical effects of trazodone.

References

CHANG, C. C.: A sensitive method for spectrophotofluorometric assay of catecholamines. Int. J. Neuropharmacol. *3:* 643–649 (1964).

JACOBS, B. L. and MCGINTY, D. J.: Effects of food deprivation on sleep and wakefulness in the rat. Exp. Neurol. *30:* 212–222 (1971).

KANEKO, T. and YAMATSU, K.: Unpublished results (1972).

KHAZAN, N. and BROWN, P.: Differential effects of three tricyclic antidepressants on sleep and REM sleep in the rat. Life Sci. *9:* 279–284 (1970).

MILLER, F. P.; COX, R. H.; SNODGRASS, W. R., and MAICKEL, R. P.: Comparative effects of *p*-chlorophenylalanine, *p*-chloroamphetamine and *p*-chloro-N-methylamphetamine on rat brain norepinephrine, serotonin and 5-hydroxyindazole-3-acetic acid. Biochem. Pharmacol. *19:* 435–442 (1970).

SILVESTRINI, B.; CIOLI, V.; BURBERI, S., and CATANESE, B.: Pharmacological properties of AF 1161, a new psychotropic drug. Int. J. Neuropharmacol. *7:* 587–599 (1968).

SILVESTRINI, B. and QUADRI, E.: Investigations on the specificity of the so-called analgesic activity of non-narcotic drugs. Europ. J. Pharmacol. *12:* 231–235 (1970).

YAMATSU, K.; KITAHARA, A.; TATENO, T.; NAKANO, S., and OHTAKE, S.: Unpublished results (1972).

YAMATSU, K. and KANEKO, T.: Abstracts of Conferences. Folia pharmac. jap. *69:* 14 (1973).

Author's address: Dr. K. YAMATSU, Department of Pharmacology, Section of Experimental Therapeutic Research, Research and Development Division, Eisai Co. Ltd., *Tokyo* (Japan)

Trazodone. Mod. Probl. Pharmacopsychiat., vol. 9, pp. 18–28,
ed. Th. A. Ban, Montreal, Que., and B. Silvestrini, Rome (Karger, Basel 1974)

Pharmacological and Biochemical Features of Trazodone

J. R. Boissier, E. Portmann-Cristesco, P. Soubrié and J. Fichelle

Institut National de la Santé et de la Recherche Médicale, Unité de Recherches de Neuro-Psycho-Pharmacologie, Paris

I wish to state before anything else that I am in full agreement with what has been said by my friend Prof. V. Longo. I particularly agree with him on the issue of the great difficulty of making any progress in psychopharmacology if we remain within the framework of presently available categories.

This methodology leads to nothing really new and it is only by giving new psychopharmacological profiles to the molecular structures that we may hope to find 'something truly new'.

As far as trazodone goes, I shall herewith present the results obtained in our laboratories.

Acute Toxicity

It appears imperative to keep in mind the LD_{50} of trazodone in order to obtain a better evaluation of its specific pharmacological activity.

With the strains of animals employed in our studies, the following LD_{50}s have been determined:

Table I

LD_{50}	Mouse	Rat
Intravenous	90 (77.5–104)	68 (60.7–76.2)
Intraperitoneal	230 (213–247)	110 (94–127)
Oral	925 (777–1,100)	500 (434–575)

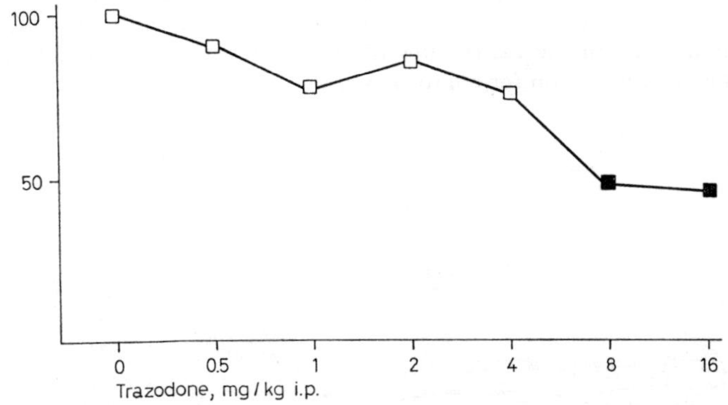

Fig. 1. Motility in the mouse (groups of 12). 30 min after trazodone – measurement during 10 min. Black squares: significant difference at $p < 0.01$.

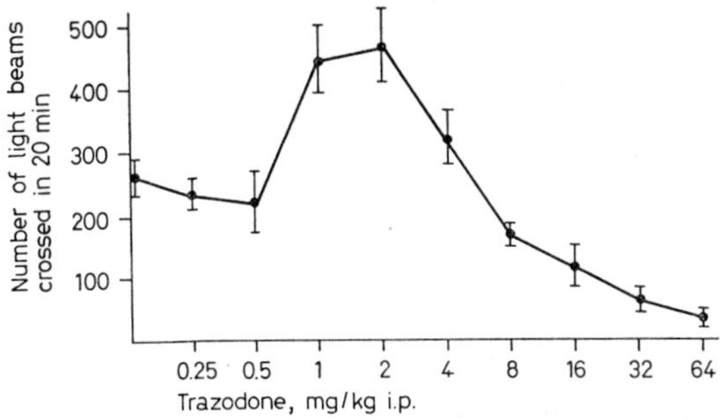

Fig. 2. Motility in the mouse (groups of 12). 30 min after trazodone – measurement during 20 min. Significant difference for 1, 2 mg/kg ($p < 0.01$) and 4 mg/kg ($p < 0.05$).

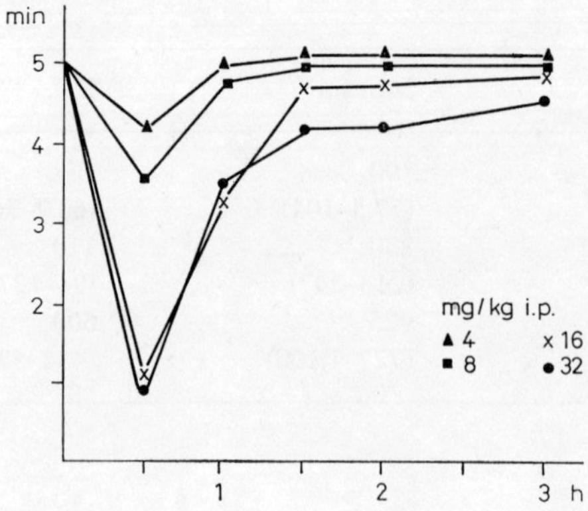

Fig. 3. Rota-rod test in the rat (groups of 10) after trazodone administration. Mean time on the step (maximum for controls: 5 min).

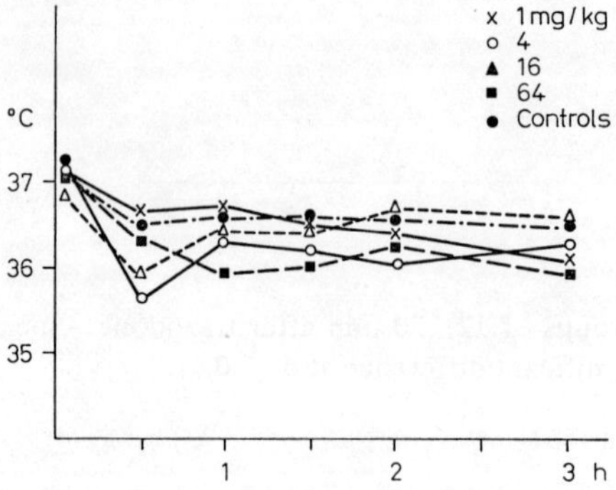

Fig. 4. Action of trazodone on rectal temperature in the mouse (groups of 12).

Psychotropic Action

1. Motility

The motility in mice has been studied with the technique which utilizes enclosures with two perpendicular light beams.

When trazodone is given i. p. 10 min prior to the beginning of the test, which lasts for a period of 30 min, a decrease in the motility is observed beginning at the dose of 8 mg/kg (fig. 1).

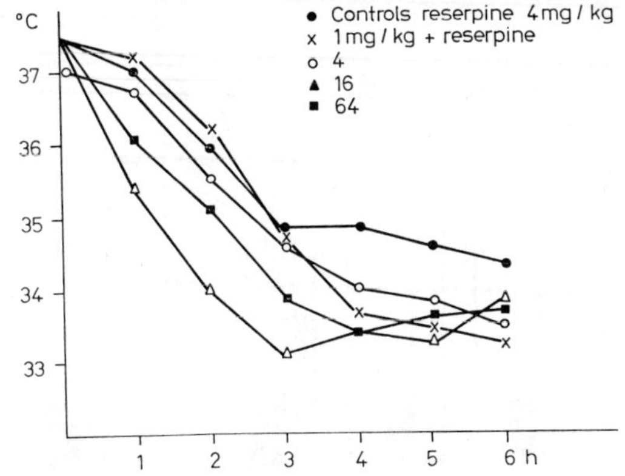

Fig. 5. Action of trazodone on reserpine-induced hypothermia in the mouse (groups of 12).

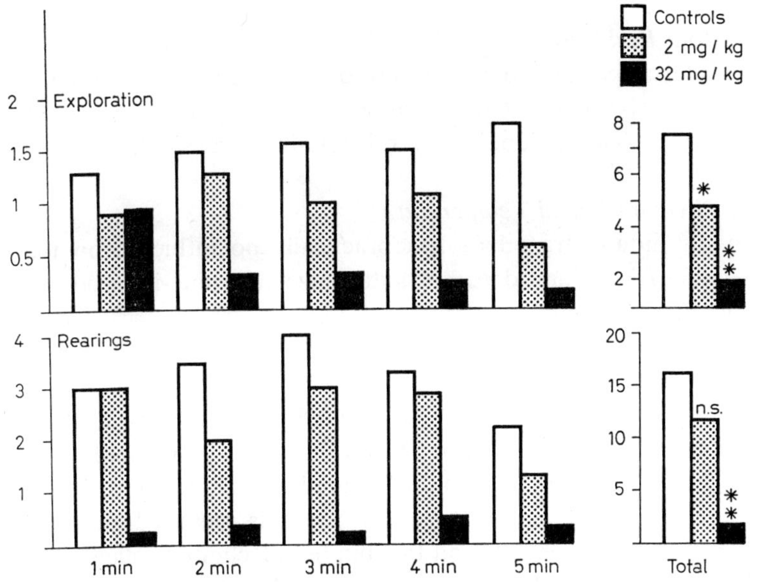

Fig. 6. Action of trazodone on the number of squares crossed in the open field in rats (groups of 12). ˣ $p < 0.01$.

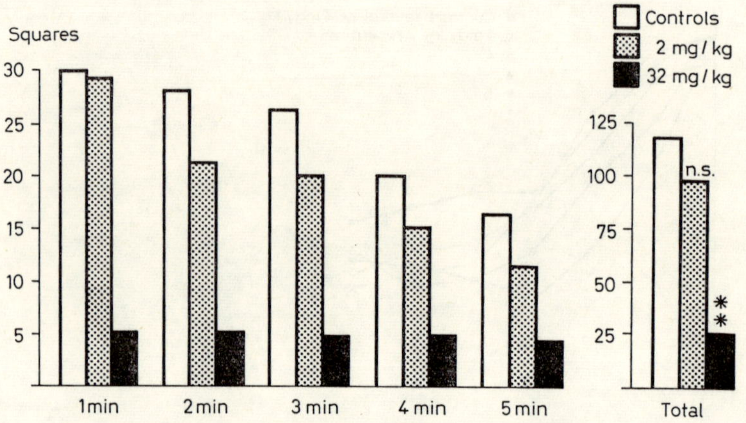

Fig. 7. Action of trazodone on exploration and rightings in the open field in rats (groups of 12). x $p < 0.05$; xx $p < 0.01$.

If the measurements are taken for a period of 20 min an increase in the motility is observed at dosages comprised between 1 and 4 mg/kg (fig. 2).

2. Rota-Rod Test

This test is performed with groups of 10 male rats. Beginning from the 4 mg/kg level a marked psychomotor incapacity is observed at about 30 min (fig. 3). This action, however, is relatively transient.

3. Effect on Rectal Temperature

In the mouse, trazodone has practically no influence on the rectal temperature (fig. 4) and does not antagonize reserpine-induced hypothermia (fig. 5).

4. Open Field

A square open field (1×1 m) painted white was used. 10×10 cm squares were drawn on the floor and on these four poles were placed with the purpose of studying the explorative ability of the animals. The number of squares crossed during a period of 5 min is recorded along with the number of explored objects and the number of climbing stands in groups of 12 male rats (fig. 6, 7). At a dose of 2 mg/kg of trazodone a significant decrease in the number of explorations was observed. All recorded parameters are significantly decreased at the 32 mg/kg dosage.

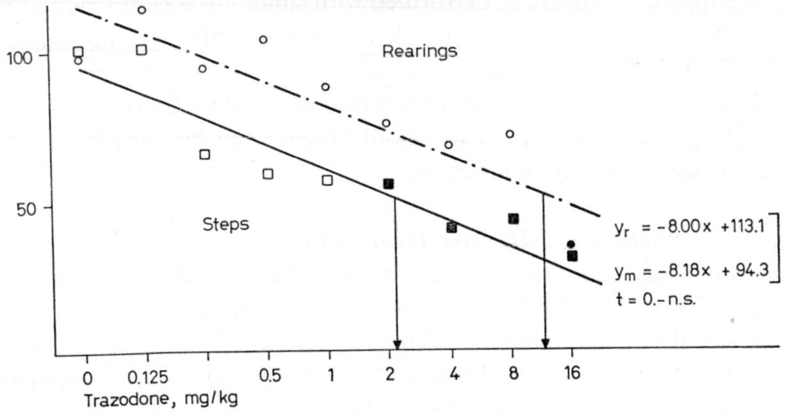

Fig. 8. Staircase test (groups of 12 rats). Black squares and circles: significant difference (0.05 < p < 0.01).

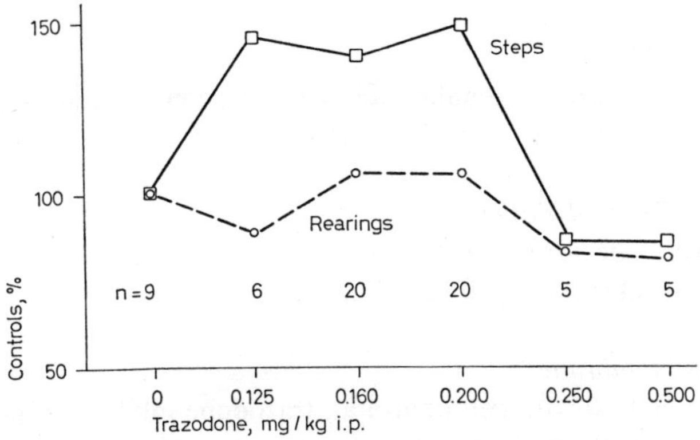

Fig. 9. Staircase test (groups of 24 rats). Significant difference (p < 0.05) at 0.125, 0.160 and 0.200 mg/kg.

5. Staircase Test

This test utilizes an enclosure where a staircase of 6 steps, each 6 cm high and of equal width, has been placed. The rats are placed one by one in the enclosure (12 rat groups are used) and the number of rightings is determined along with the number of steps climbed during the 5-min period.

Trazodone reduces simultaneously and equally both the rightings and the number of steps climbed (fig. 8).

A supplementary study performed with small doses of trazodone shows that between 0.125 and 0.200 mg/kg, trazodone increases the number of steps climbed (fig. 9).

If we compare these results with those obtained with oxazepam (fig. 10) and chlorpromazine (fig. 11) we should favour the hypothesis that trazodone possesses an anxiolytic action.

6. Potentiation of 5-Hydroxytryptophane

Convulsions and tremors are induced by 5-HTP in rats previously treated with an MAO inhibitor. These convulsions are prolonged in time when trazodone at amounts superior to 32 mg/kg is administered i. p. prior to 5-HTP. Animals previously treated with pargyline display greater toxicity to L-dopa when they received trazodone at doses of 1–8 mg/kg.

Adrenolytic Action

1. Isolated Rabbit Ear

Trazodone antagonizes adrenaline-induced vasoconstriction. The inhibiting dose/50 is around 14 μg/ml (fig. 12).

2. Guinea Pig Seminal Vesicle

The effective concentration/50 capable of inhibiting up to 50% adrenaline-induced submaximal contraction is near 1.10^{-7}.

3. Nictitating Membrane

In cats anaesthetized with pentobarbital, trazodone inhibits (1 mg/kg, i. v.) the contraction of the nictitating membrane induced by noradrenaline, adrenaline and 5-hydroxytryptamine. The adrenolytic action does not give rise to moderate sympatholytic and ganglioplegic actions except at doses 30 times higher (fig. 13).

4. Arterial Pressure in the Dog

Adrenaline-induced hypertension is inhibited at 50% following i. v. injection of 0.1 mg/kg of trazodone. The same applies to noradrenaline-induced hypertension. A complete adrenolytic action is obtained with trazodone doses of between 3 and 10 mg/kg. Isoprenaline-induced hypotension is slightly decreased following 10 mg/kg injection of trazodone.

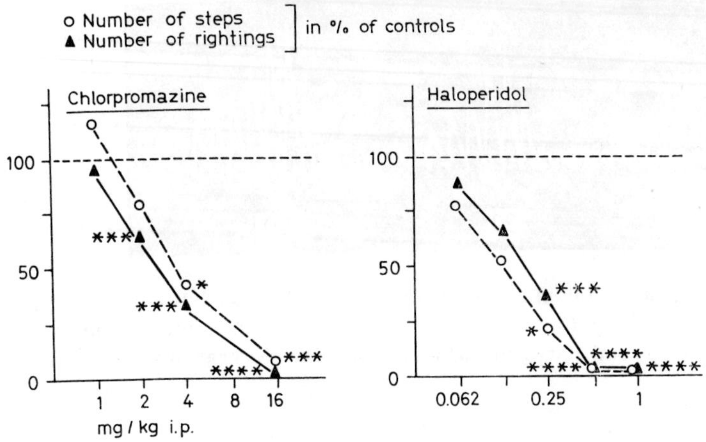

Fig. 10. Staircase test (groups of 24 rats). Action of chlorpromazine and haloperidol.

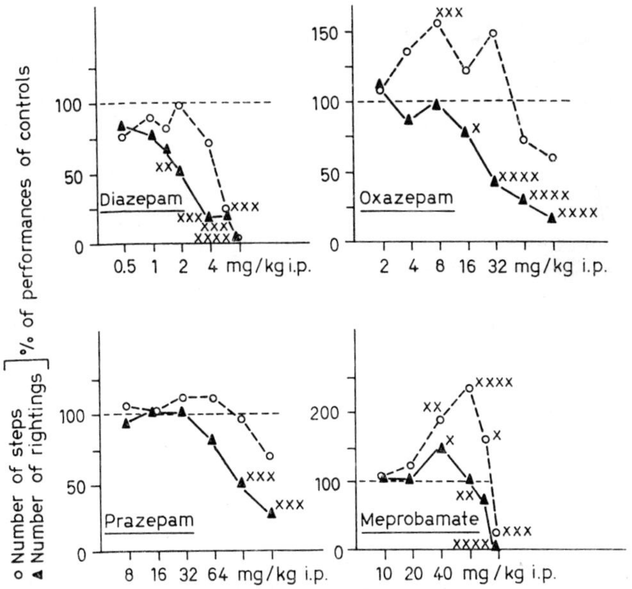

Fig. 11. Staircase test (groups auf 24 rats). Action of benzodiazepines and meprobamate.

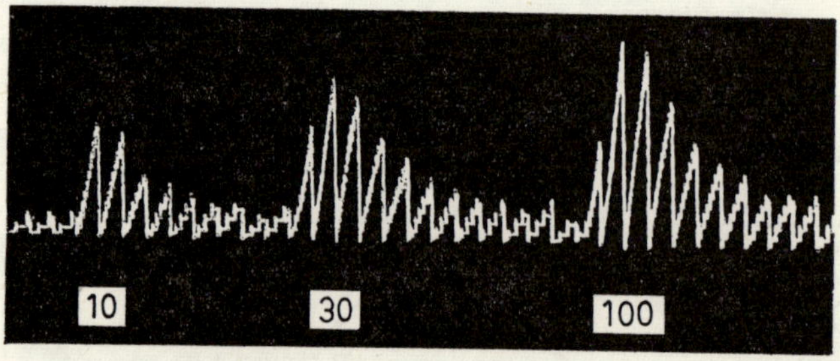

Fig. 12. Isolated rabbit ear. Perfusion of a McEwan solution at 1.10^{-7} of adrenaline. Fleish recording drop outflow impulse counter (30-sec interval timer). Injection in circuit of 10, 30 and 100 μg of trazodone provokes blockage of vasoconstriction.

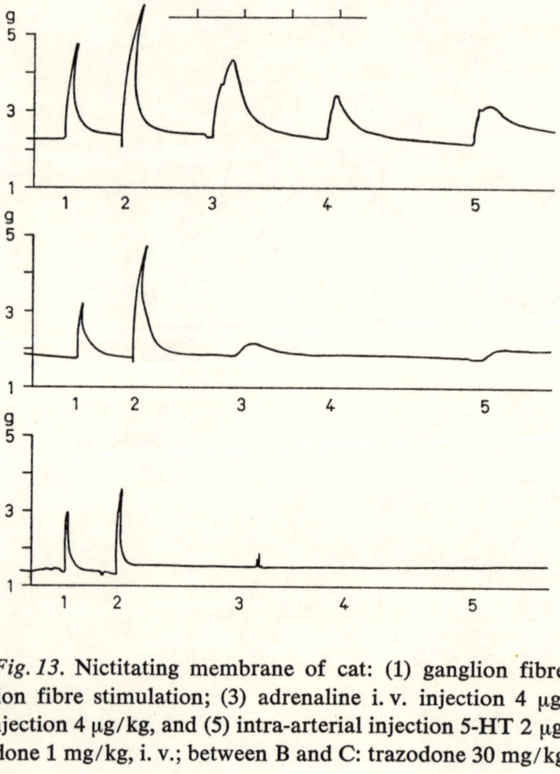

Fig. 13. Nictitating membrane of cat: (1) ganglion fibre stimulation; (2) postganglion fibre stimulation; (3) adrenaline i. v. injection 4 μg/kg; (4) noradrenaline i. v. injection 4 μg/kg, and (5) intra-arterial injection 5-HT 2 μg/kg. Between A and B: trazodone 1 mg/kg, i. v.; between B and C: trazodone 30 mg/kg, i. v.

Table II

Fractions	Weight fractions, mg	Dopamine, ng/g	Noradrenaline, ng/g	5-HT, ng/g
Limbic cortex				
Control	750 ± 57.2	356.60 ± 27.97	305.34 ± 49.42	346.68 ± 72.85
Treated	1,033 ± 30.5	110.57	317.43 ± 28.82	404.90 ± 65.02
Septum				
Control	322 ± 22.7	1,105.61 ± 81.01	375.67 ± 47.74	974.54 ± 241.31
Treated	340 ± 6.5	465.78 ± 109.55	497.28 ± 24.55	668.52 ± 128.50
Amygdala				
Control	423 ± 20.5	272.50 ± 84.89	520.31 ± 26.80	1,126.15 ± 39.54
Treated	457 ± 30.4	318.08 ± 127.32	471.05 ± 91.25	804.15 ± 10.87[1]
Hippocampus				
Control	939 ± 71.0	34.64 ± 15.28	249.41 ± 37.19	348.78
Treated	1,029 ± 33.3	175.63 ± 26.12[2]	239.54 ± 16.17	350.89 ± 23.75

1 $p < 0.01$
2 $p < 0.02$

Cerebral Biochemistry

A limited study has been performed with rats in this direction. Trazodone was administered at the dosage of 8 mg/kg i. p., and 30 min later the animals were decapitated. The brain was extracted within 15 sec and was slowly frozen in liquid nitrogen.

Sagittal slices of 0.8 mm were obtained with a microtone for the main structures, i. e. limbic system, limbic cortex, septum, amygdala and hippocampus. The results obtained are shown in table II.

Conclusion

The results obtained are not easy to interpret in the light of the previsional psychopharmacology as we defined it.

However, trazodone seems to be endowed, at low doses, with an anxiolytic action which, at higher doses, is masked by a psychosedative action.

Trazodone does not possess the psychopharmacological profile of tricyclic antidepressants. It is not anticataleptic, not an antireserpine substance, and does not potentiate noradrenaline. On the other hand, TRH does not possess these properties either, while it potentiates 5-HTP like trazodone. Therefore, one cannot exclude the possibility of an antidepressant action of trazodone.

Trazodone possesses a marked adrenolytic action, although it is not possible to establish yet whether this property can play a role in its clinical activity. The pharmacological profile of trazodone, unusual as it is, justifies the extensive clinical investigations.

References

BOISSIER, J. R. et SIMON, P.: Dissociation de deux composantes dans le comportement d'investigation de la souris. Arch. int. Pharmacodyn. *147:* 372–387 (1964).

BOISSIER, J. R.: Situation libre et psychotropes; in Symp. Pharmacology of Conditioning, Learning and Retention, pp. 25–46 (Pergamon Press, London 1965).

BOISSIER, J. R. and SIMON, P.: Evaluation of experimental technique in the psychopharmacology of emotion. Ann. N. Y. Acad. Sci. *159:* 898–914 (1969).

BOISSIER, J .R.; ZEBROWSKA-LUPINA, I., et SIMON, P.: Profil pharmacologique du prazépam. Arch. int. Pharmacodyn. *196:* 330–344 (1972).

SIMON, P.: Les anxiolytiques: possibilité d'étude chez l'animal. Actualités pharmacol. *23:* 47–78 (1970).

SOUBRIE, P.: Open-field chez le rat; inter-relation entre locomotion, exploration et émotivité. J. Pharmacol. *2:* 457–472 (1971).

SOUBRIE, P. et BOISSIER, J. R.: Redressements et comportement exploratoire chez le rat. C. R. Acad. Sci. *274:* 2534–2536 (1972).

THIEBOT, M. H.; SOUBRIE, P.; SIMON, P. et BOISSIER, J. R.: Dissociation de deux composantes du comportement chez le rat sous l'effet de psychotropes. Application à l'étude des anxiolytiques. Psychopharmacologia, Berl. *31:* 77–90 (1973).

Author's address: Prof. J. R. BOISSIER, Unité de Neuropsychopharmacologie de l'INSERM, 2, Rue d'Alésia, *F-75014 Paris* (France)

Trazodone. Mod. Probl. Pharmacopsychiat., vol. 9, pp. 29–46,
ed. Th. A. Ban, Montreal, Que., and B. Silvestrini, Rome (Karger, Basel 1974)

Biochemical Studies with Trazodone

A New Psychoactive Drug

S. GARATTINI

Istituto di Ricerche Farmacologiche 'Mario Negri', Milano

Introduction

Trazodone, 2-{3-[4(m-chlorophenyl) 1-piperazinyl]-propyl}-s-triazolo [4, 3-a]-pirydin-3-(2H) one, is a new psychoactive drug [SILVESTRINI *et al.*, 1968; BAIOCCHI *et al.*, 1973 a; PALAZZO, 1973; SILVESTRINI and LISCIANI, 1973], showing a therapeutical effect in several pathological conditions, including anxiety and endogenous depressions [DE GREGORIO and DIONISIO, 1971; UCHA UDABE, 1973; BAN and LEHMANN, 1973; NAIR *et al.*, 1973; AMIN *et al.*, 1973; KNOBEL, 1973; ANTONELLI *et al.*, 1973]. However, it is difficult to place it into one of the classes of drugs acting on the central nervous system. In fact, trazodone does not show monoamine oxidase (MAO) inhibition [CONSOLO, unpublished observations], it does not possess the pharmacological profile of the tricyclic antidepressant agents (antagonism toward reserpine, potentiation of L-dopa, increase of adrenergic activity), nor does it show the characteristics of reserpine-like agents [LONGO and SCOTTI DE CAROLIS, 1973]. Furthermore, trazodone does not exhibit any stimulant effects and does not present neuroleptic properties (cataleptogenic effect, antagonism toward amphetamine and apomorphine).

However, it shares with the phenothiazines a strong antiserotonin effect (bronchial spasm) *in vivo* [SILVESTRINI *et al.*, 1968] and isolated stomach of rat *in vitro* [KANEKO and YAMATSU, 1972], and the capacity to inhibit the response to painful and unpleasant stimuli [SILVESTRINI and QUADRI,

1 The experimental work quoted in this review has been carried out by Drs. S. BAREGGI (noradrenaline); A. FRIGERIO (metabolism); A. JORI (dopamine); H. LADINSKY (acetylcholine); M. SALMONA (aminoacids); R. SAMANIN (serotonin).

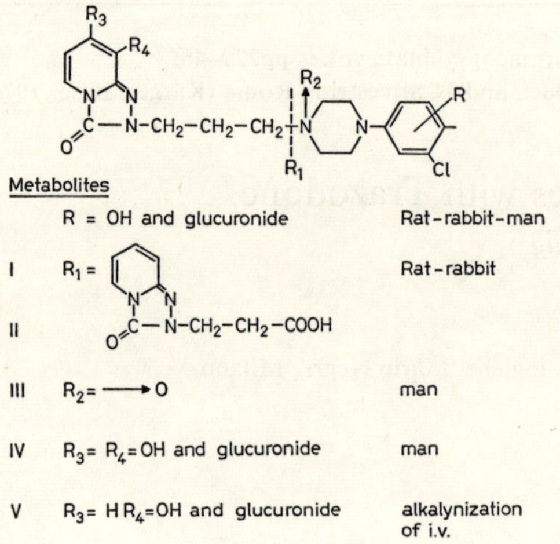

Fig. 1. Metabolic transformation of trazodone. Other metabolites have been suggested, but are not yet identified.

1970; YAMATSU *et al.*, 1973]. This report intends to deal primarily with the biochemical pharmacology of this drug, i. e. metabolic transformation, pharmacokinetic aspects and interactions with putative chemical transmitters in the brain.

Metabolism of Trazodone

Trazodone is extensively transformed in the body since only a small fraction of the administered dose is excreted as such in the urine and feces of both experimental animals and man [CATANESE and LISCIANI, 1970; YAMATO *et al.*, 1973].

As depicted in figure 1, the metabolism of trazodone may follow several biochemical pathways. BAIOCCHI *et al.* [1973 b] separated, by thin-layer chromatography, a N-oxide derivative, which was identified by several chemico-physical techniques and by the availability of the synthetic compound.

YAMATO *et al.* [1973], who used trazodone labelled with ^{14}C in the triazole ring in their studies, have described a splitting of the molecule which, by oxidation, gives rise to oxo-triazolepyridinpropionic acid (TPA).

This compound has been isolated both in a free and a conjugated form from rat urine.

Several hydroxylated derivatives, excreted in the urine of rats and man as glucuronide conjugates, have also been characterized. For instance, a diol derivative in the pyridine ring has been isolated and identified by mass spectrometry and nuclear magnetic resonance (NMR) techniques [BAIOCCHI *et al.*, 1973]. The mechanism of formation of this dihydroxy metabolite is not yet known, and it would be interesting to establish whether this requires the presence of an intermediate epoxide. The monohydroxy derivative is also present in human urine, but it may be formed from the diol in alkalyne conditions [BAIOCCHI *et al.*, 1973 b].

A hydroxyl derivate in the phenyl ring has been described both by YAMATO *et al.* [1973] and BAIOCCHI *et al.* [1973 b]. The position of the hydroxyl groups has not yet been unequivocally established. The only possibility which was excluded is that the hydroxylation occurs in position para in respect to the chlorine atom.

The time course of the pharmacological effects does not suggest the presence of active metabolites.

Pharmacokinetic Aspects

As already mentioned, a very small percentage of trazodone in its original form is excreted in the urine. For instance, in rats, after the oral administration of 4 mg/kg of labelled trazodone, only less than 3 % of the administered dose is excreted as such in urine [FUJITA *et al.*, 1973; YAMATO *et al.*, 1973].

Similar results have been obtained in rats and in man by CATANESE and LISCIANI [1970]. The levels of trazodone in plasma and in tissues have been measured in two ways: (1) spectrofluorometrically [CATANESE and LISCIANI, 1970], and (2) by employing ^{14}C-labelled compound [FUJITA *et al.*, 1973; YAMATO *et al.*, 1973]. With both these methods the identity of trazodone has been checked by using thin layer chromatography. When the experimental conditions were comparable, the two methods gave substantially similar results. It should, however, be recalled that the methods used have not been unequivocally controlled for their specificity in measuring only trazodone.

In rats, trazodone is absorbed very rapidly when administered by the oral route [YAMATO *et al.*, 1973; FUJITA *et al.*, 1973]. In dogs the absorption

Table I. Effect of trazodone on acetylcholine and choline levels in discrete areas of the rat brain

Brain area	Acetylcholine, μg/g ± SE		Choline, μg/g ± SE	
	saline	trazodone	saline	trazodone
Hemispheres	2.05 ± 0.07	2.29 ± 0.09	6.15 ± 0.11	6.00 ± 0.15
Diencephalon	2.89 ± 0.07	2.66 ± 0.11	6.54 ± 0.14	6.40 ± 0.11
Mesencephalon	2.47 ± 0.10	2.32 ± 0.08	7.20 ± 0.22	7.81 ± 0.17

Trazodone was given at a dose of 50 mg/kg i. p. and determinations were carried out 1 h after drug administration. Acetylcholine and choline were determined by the radioisotopic method of SAELENS *et al.* [1970].

Table II. Effect of trazodone on brain dopamine and striatum homovanillic acid (HVA) in rats

Time, min	HVA/μg/g ± SE	DA (μg/g) ± SE	HVA (μg/g) ± SE	DA (μg/g) ± SE
	trazodone, 50 mg/kg i. p.		trazodone, 25 mg/kg i. p.	
0	218 ± 18	10.5 ± 0.5	–	9.8 ± 0.2
30	257 ± 32	–	–	–
60	114 ± 3[1]	5.5 ± 0.3[1]	157 ± 8[1]	7.7 ± 0.1[1]
120	166 ± 6[1]	6.7 ± 0.1[1]	247 ± 8	8.5 ± 0.3

1 $p < 0.01$.
Dopamine was measured according to CHANG [1964]; TAYLOR and LAVERTY [1969]. HVA according to KORF *et al.* [1971].

is, instead, relatively slow [CATANESE and LISCIANI, 1970]. The disappearance of trazodone from plasma is also more rapid in rats than in dogs or in man. A study is now in progress to investigate in detail the pharmacokinetic parameters of trazodone.

Little is known about the tissue distribution of trazodone. This compound does not specifically accumulate in brain, but it concentrates in liver and in kidneys [YAMATO *et al.*, 1973]. More studies are, however, required to establish any selective localization of trazodone.

Table III. Effect of trazodone on levels and turnover of dopamine in the rat striatum

Treatment, mg/kg i. p. × 5 days	Striatum dopamine, μg/g ± SE	Rate of dis-appearance, Kh^{-1} ± SE	Turnover rate, μg/g/h	Turnover time, h
Saline	10.3 ± 0.4	0.36 ± 0.003	3.71	2.8
Trazodone 50	7.3 ± 0.2[1]	0.38 ± 0.03	2.78	2.6

1 $p < 0.01$. The levels of striatum dopamine have been measured according to CHANG [1964]; TAYLOR and LAVERTY [1969].
The rate of dopamine disappearance was established by measuring striatum dopamine before and 1, 2 and 4 h after administration of α-methyltyrosine methyl ester (200 mg/kg i. v.). The last dose of trazodone was given 2 h before the experiment.

Interactions with Brain Acetylcholine

The effect of trazodone on brain acetylcholine and choline in rats has been studied 1 h after its oral administration (50 mg/kg). The results obtained (table I) concern the levels of choline and acetylcholine in the diencephalon, mesencephalon and hemispheres. No substantial changes have been observed. In contrast, previous studies have indicated that benzodiazepines and barbiturates [CONSOLO *et al.*, 1972], but not chlorpromazine or imipramine, increase the levels of brain acetylcholine, probably in relation to their sedative effect.

Interactions with Brain Dopamine

Trazodone, at doses of 25 and 50 mg/kg, induces a slight decrease in brain dopamine levels. This effect is more marked, in the striatum where this monoamine is selectively concentrated (table II).

However, no changes in the dopamine turnover rate were detected in the striatum when dopamine synthesis was blocked by the administration of α-methyltyrosine (table III).

Trazodone also produces a transient decrease in the levels of the major metabolite of dopamine, homovanillic acid, in the striatum.

Table IV. Effect of trazodone on brain noradrenaline in rats

Time, min	Brain noradrenaline (μg/g ± SE) after trazodone	
	25 mg/kg i. p.	50 mg/kg i. p.
0	0.36 ± 0.03	0.35 ± 0.01
30	0.32 ± 0.01	0.26 ± 0.01[1]
60	0.32 ± 0.01	0.27 ± 0.01[1]
120	0.34 ± 0.02	0.32 ± 0.01

1 $p < 0.01$.
Brain noradrenaline was measured according to the method of HÄGGENDAL [1963].

These data are quite different from those obtained with classic neuroleptics, such as chlorpromazine or haloperidol. In fact, these two drugs, which are considered inhibitors of dopaminergic receptors, increase the level of homovanillic acid and the turnover of dopamine in the striatum [DA PRADA and PLETSCHER, 1966]. On the other hand, tricyclic antidepressant agents are considered to have no effect on the metabolism of dopamine. Some drugs known to lower the concentrations of homovanillic acid in the striatum are the dopaminergic stimulants, such as apomorphine and piribedil [GARATTINI *et al.*, 1972].

Interactions with Brain Noradrenaline

Trazodone decreases the levels of brain noradrenaline in rats (table IV). This effect is particularly evident in the brain stem and in the telencephalon (table V).

In the rat brain, the reduction in noradrenaline is not accompanied by any change in the major metabolite of this catecholamine, namely MHPG-sulphate [SCHANBERG *et al.*, 1968]. However, an increase of this metabolite, after inhibiting its transport by probenecid, is more evident for trazodone-treated than for control rats (fig. 2).

In order to obtain more information on the mechanism responsible for the action of trazodone on catecholamines, a study on the uptake of brain noradrenaline has been carried out. Noradrenaline was injected intraven-

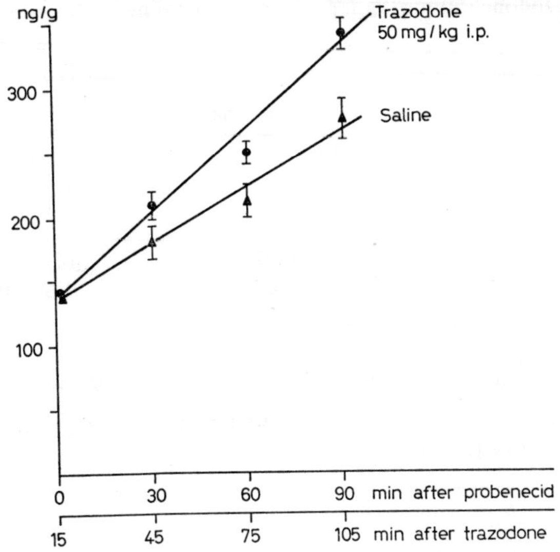

Fig. 2. Levels of MHPG-sulphate on rat brain after trazodone (50 mg/kg i. p.) in combination with probenecid (400 mg/kg i. p.). Brain MHPG-SO_4 was measured according to MEEK and NEFF [1973].

ticularly before or after the administration of trazodone; in both cases, a slight inhibition of the accumulation of noradrenaline in the whole brain was evident (table VI).

In another experiment, it was established that the effect of trazodone on the accumulation of noradrenaline is confined to the brain stem (table VII). Similarly to desipramine, the inhibition of noradrenaline accumulation is accompanied by an increase of normetanephrine, without any change in the deaminated acid metabolites (table VIII). It is also evident from table VIII, that the effect of trazodone on the metabolism of noradrenaline is different from that exerted by reserpine.

Interactions with Heart Noradrenaline

Since it has been suggested that the inhibition of catecholamines in the heart may be a factor in the cardiotoxicity exerted by tricyclic antidepressant agents, particularly in elderly subjects, it was decided to study the effect of trazodone on heart catecholamines. The experiment was carried out *in*

Table V. Effect of trazodone (50 mg/kg i. p.) on noradrenaline in discrete areas of rat brain

Brain area	Noradrenaline, µg/g ± SE	
	saline	trazodone
Brain stem	0.70 ± 0.05	0.50 ± 0.05[1]
Telediencephalon	0.35 ± 0.02	0.27 ± 0.01[2]
Hypothalamus	1.80 ± 0.08	1.60 ± 0.01

1 $p < 0.05$.
2 $p < 0.01$.
The determinations were carried out 1 h after drug administration according to the method of HÄGGENDAL [1963].

Table VI. Effect of trazodone on the uptake of brain noradrenaline

Treatment, mg/kg i. p.	Brain noradrenaline	
	^{3}H-NA, ng/g ± SD	^{3}H-NA, % total radioactivity
Saline	28 ± 4	66
Trazodone 50 (1 h after ^{3}H-NA)	20 ± 1[1]	44
Trazodone 50 (1 h before ^{3}H-NA)	23 ± 1[1]	56

1 $p < 0.05$.
^{3}H-NA was injected into lateral ventricle (1µg; 3.7 µCi) 4 h before sacrifice.

vitro, by using isolated rat atria and following the uptake of ^{3}H-labelled noradrenaline added to the medium. Table IX shows that trazodone inhibits noradrenaline uptake only at relatively high concentrations, which are unlikely to occur *in vivo*.

Conversely, several antidepressant agents exert a clear inhibition at doses which are in a range of 100–1,000 times lower than those used for

Table VII. Effect of trazodone on the uptake of brain ^{3}H-noradrenaline injected into the lateral ventricle

Brain area	^{3}H-Noradrenaline, ng/g ± SD		
	saline	trazodone, 25 mg/kg i. p.	trazodone, 50 mg/kg i. p.
Brain stem	10±1	9±1	6±2[1]
Diencephalon	6±2	6±1	4±2
Telencephalon	1±0.6	1±0.4	1±0.4
Striatum	5±1	5±1	5±1

1 $p < 0.05$.
For details see table VIII.

Table VIII. Effect of various drugs on the uptake of brain noradrenaline

Treatment	Dose, mg/kg i. p.	Time, min	Brain, % total radioactivity		
			^{3}H-NA	^{3}H-NM	^{3}H-deaminated metabolites
Saline		–	56± 6	4±1	40±3
Trazodone	50	30	36±13[1]	10±4[1]	42±4
Desipramine	20	60	31±11[1]	11±3[1]	40±1
Amphetamine	20	60	20± 6[1]	8±2[1]	51±3
Reserpine	5	120	7±10[1]	2±1[1]	71±8[1]

1 ^{3}H-NA into the lateral ventricle as in table VIII. NM = normetanephrine.

trazodone. During these observations, another effect of trazodone became evident, namely its capacity to release noradrenaline from the atria; a phenomenon similar to that which occurs in the case of tyramine.

The decrease of atrial noradrenaline and the increased radioactivity in the medium, after addition of trazodone or tyramine, are presented in table X.

Table IX. Effect of trazodone and other tricyclic antidepressant agents on the uptake of 1-^{3}H-noradrenaline in isolated rat atria

Drug	ED_{50}, molar
Trazodone	3.6×10^{-5}
Imipramine	4.5×10^{-7}
Desipramine	1.3×10^{-8}
Amitriptyline	4.2×10^{-7}
Nortriptyline	8.1×10^{-8}
Doxepin	5×10^{-7}
Desmethyl-doxepin	5×10^{-8}

Table X. Effect of trazodone and tyramine on the release of ^{3}H-noradrenaline from rat atria

Drug added, g/l	^{3}H-NA in atria after 2 h, DPM/g	^{3}H-NA in medium after 2 h, $\times 10^5$ DPM
Saline	9,000	165
Trazodone 10^{-5}	6,600	305
Tyramine 10^{-6}	2,800	465

Table XI. Effect of trazodone on the levels of brain 5HT and 5HIAA in rats

Time, min	Brain levels (μg/g $\pm$ SE) after trazodone			
	25 mg/kg		50 mg/kg	
	5HT	5HIAA	5HT	5HIAA
0	0.32	0.26	0.31	0.25
30	0.33	0.27	0.33	0.28
60	0.36[1]	0.25	0.36[1]	0.28
120	0.37[2]	0.25	0.34	0.25

1 $p < 0.05$.
2 $p < 0.01$.
The biochemical determinations were performed according to the method of GIACALONE and VALZELLI [1969].

Table XII. Effect of trazodone on the levels of serotonin (5HT) in discrete brain areas of rats

Brain area	5HT, ng/g ± SE	
	saline	trazodone
Brain stem	0.33 ± 0.08	0.36 ± 0.09
Telediencephalon	0.17 ± 0.05	0.15 ± 0.01
Hypothalamus	1.70 ± 0.60	2.40 ± 0.60

Table XIII. Levels of brain 5HT and 5HIAA after treatment with trazodone (50 mg/kg i. p.) in rats pretreated with pargyline (75 mg/kg i. p.)

Time, min	Brain levels, μg/g ± SE			
	controls		trazodone	
	5HT	5HIAA	5HT	5HIAA
0	0.32 ± 0.01	0.26 ± 0.01	0.35 ± 0.02	0.28 ± 0.01
15	0.37 ± 0.02	0.15 ± 0.01	0.41 ± 0.01	0.20 ± 0.01
30	0.48 ± 0.02	0.12 ± 0.01	0.50 ± 0.01	0.17 ± 0.01
60	0.53 ± 0.02	0.11 ± 0.01	0.53 ± 0.03	0.12 ± 0.01

Levels of brain 5HT and 5HIAA were measured according to the method of GIACALONE and VALZELLI [1969].

Interactions with Brain Serotonin

Previous studies have indicated that trazodone is an effective anti-serotonin agent in various peripheral preparations [KANEKO and YAMATSU, 1972; SILVESTRINI *et al.*, 1968] while it increases the central effects of 5-hydroxytryptophan [LONGO and SCOTTI DE CAROLIS, 1973]. Trazodone, even at high doses, produces only a marginal effect on the concentration of brain serotonin (5HT) and 5-hydroxyindolacetic acid (5HIAA), as reported in table XI. YAMATSU *et al.* [1973] have found a decrease in brain 5HIAA by trazodone, but only at doses (160 mg/kg) which resulted in

Table XIV. Effect of trazodone and of several tricyclic antidepressant drugs on the depletion of brain 5HT produced by fenfluramine on rats

Treatment	Dose, mg/kg i. p.	5HT Brain level, μg/g ± SE
Saline		0.34 ± 0.01
Fenfluramine	15	0.13 ± 0.01[1]
Trazodone	25	
Fenfluramine	15	0.25 ± 0.03[2]
Trazodone	12.5	
Fenfluramine	15	0.24 ± 0.01[2]
Trazodone	6.2	
Fenfluramine	15	0.24 ± 0.02[2]
Cl-Imipramine	10	
Fenfluramine	15	0.23 ± 0.02[2]
Imipramine	10	
Fenfluramine	15	0.17 ± 0.01
Desipramine	10	
Fenfluramine	15	0.18 ± 0.02

1 $p < 0.01$ in respect to saline.
2 $p < 0.01$ in respect to fenfluramine.
Trazodone or other drugs were given 30 min before fenfluramine. Animals were sacrificed 2 h after fenfluramine.

marked neurological symptoms. A decrease in brain 5HIAA has also been reported by ANGELUCCI [1973], when 25 mg/kg of trazodone were administered. The discrepancy shown by the data of the latter author may be related to the basal levels of brain 5HT, which are substantially higher than in these results. In any case, it seems remarkable that the decrease in 5HT and 5HIAA in the mouse brain, which was observed by ANGELUCCI [1973], occurred at relatively low doses.

Further studies were carried out by measuring 5HT in various rat brain areas (hypothalamus, brain stem and telediencephalon) but also in this case trazodone, at the dose of 50 mg/kg i. p., proved to be inactive (table XII).

A repeated treatment with trazodone in rats (50 mg/kg i. p. × 7 days) did not change the levels of brain 5HT and 5HIAA when the determinations were performed at 2 h after the last administration of this drug.

Since it is known that changes in brain 5HT turnover may occur even when the levels are normal, it was decided to approach the determinations

Table XV. Effect of trazodone on aminoacid brain levels in rats

Minutes after trazodone, 50 mg/kg i. p.	Brain		Brain	
	Aspartic acid	asparagine	glutamic acid	glutamine
0	0.439±0.02	0.734±0.01	1.635±0.04	0.407±0.02
30	0.444±0.03	0.735±0.02	1.627±0.02	0.413±0.01
60	0.433±0.01	0.735±0.02	1.632±0.01	0.411±0.01
120	0.438±0.01	0.746±0.04	1.625±0.01	0.418±0.01

Each value represents the mean (mg/g) + SE of four determinations.
Aspartic acid was measured according to BERGMEYER *et al.* [1970]; glutamic acid according to BERNT and BERGMEYER [1970]; glutamine and asparagine according to NAHORSKI [1971].

of this kinetic parameter by blocking MAO *in vivo.* The rate of increase of 5HT and the rate of decline of 5HIAA, after blockade of MAO (pargyline 75 mg/kg i. p.), can be used for calculating the rate and time of brain 5HT turnover [TOZER *et al.,* 1966]. The data reported in table XIII do not suggest any major effect of trazodone on the decline of 5HIAA or on the rise of 5HT after MAO blockade.

Another study was carried out to investigate, even in an indirect manner, the effect of trazodone on the uptake of brain 5HT. Previous investigations have shown that chlorimipramine, a known inhibitor of 5HT uptake [CARLSSON *et al.,* 1969], is able to counteract the decrease in brain 5HT, produced by fenfluramine [GHEZZI *et al.,* 1973].

This effect was not exerted by other tricyclic antidepressant agents, such as desipramine [GHEZZI *et al.,* 1973] known to inhibit noradrenaline but not serotonin uptake. The interpretation given to these results was that chlorimipramine could inhibit the uptake of fenfluramine on the serotonergic nerve terminals, therefore blocking the action of the latter drug on the 5HT stores. This hypothesis was also consistent with the finding that chlorimipramine did not alter the levels of fenfluramine in the brain [GHEZZI *et al.,* 1973], nor did it affect the action of fenfluramine on the dopaminergic system [GARATTINI 1973]. Even at relatively low doses, trazodone is also able to inhibit the depletion of brain 5HT, induced by fenfluramine in rats, as summarised in table XIV. A hypothesis on the mechanism

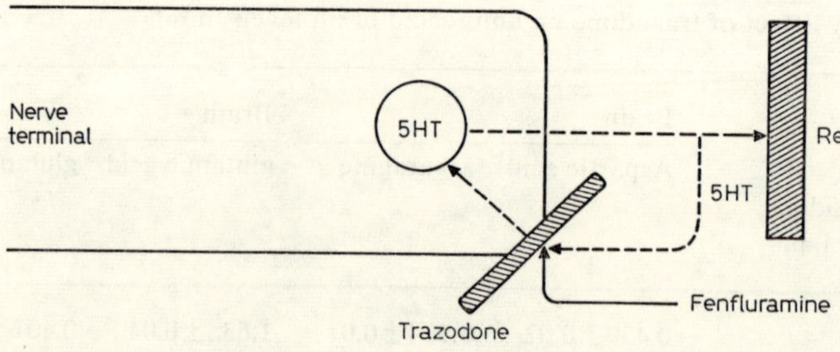

Fig. 3. Proposed mechanism of action of trazodone on brain serotonin.

of action of trazodone in this respect is depicted in figure 3. It should be stressed, however, that further studies are needed to exclude the possibility that trazodone may affect the availability of fenfluramine for the brain.

Interactions with Brain Aminoacids

In an effort to detect other neurological changes produced by trazodone, the brain levels of several aminoacids have been measured after the administration of the drug under study.

The results reported in table XV show that trazodone, at the dose of 50 mg/kg i. p., does not exert any effect on the levels of glutamic acid, aspartic acid, glutamine and asparagine in the rat brain.

Conclusions

The studies carried out with trazodone are preliminary and further experimental investigations will elucidate the distribution and the metabolism of this drug in various animal species. The same considerations may apply to the studies concerning the neurochemical changes produced by trazodone. However, one firm conclusion may already be reached, i. e. trazodone shows a neurochemical profile in regard to its action on brain monoamines which does not overlap with that of any one of the other known psychotropic drugs.

The conclusion becomes quite evident on the basis of the data shown in table XVI which summarises the effect of several drugs on the brain levels of various monoamines (acetylcholine, dopamine, noradrenaline and serotonin).

Table XVI. Comparative effects of several psychotropic drugs on brain monoamines

	Brain		Striatum			Brain			Brain			
	Ach.	choline	HVA	DA	DA turn-over	NA	MO-PEG-SO_4	NA uptake	5HT	5HIAA	5HT turn-over	5HT uptake
Diazepam	↑	—	—	—	—	—	—	—	—	—	—	—
Pentobarbital	↑	—	—	—	—	—	—	—	—	—	—	—
Reserpine	—	—	↑	↓	↑	↓	↑	↓	↓	↑	↑	↓
Chlorpromazine	—	—	↑	—	↑	—	—	—	—	—	—	—
Haloperidol[1]	—	—	↑	—	↑	—	—	—	—	—	—	—
MAO inhibitors	—	—	↓	↑		↑	↓	—	↑	↓		—
Desipramine	—	—	—	—	—	—	—	↓	—	—	—	—
Chlorimipramine			—	—	—	—	—	↓	—	—	—	↓
Amphetamine	—	—	↑	—	↑	↓		↓	—	—	—	—
Trazodone	—	—	↓	↓	—	↓	—	↓	-↓	-↓	—	↓

1 Ach increased at a high dose (4 mg/kg) but not at 1 mg/kg.

It is very difficult to correlate any one of the biochemical changes observed in the brain with the pharmacological effects of trazodone. The main group of effects seems to be related to the level of serotonin. If the inhibition of 5HT uptake really takes place in the brain, this may contribute towards explaining the increase in total sleeping time observed in animals [YAMATSU *et al.*, 1973] and in man [CASSANO *et al.*, 1973] after the administration of trazodone. This effect on brain serotonin, which is similar to that exerted by chlorimipramine, may also have a significance in regard to the peculiar type of antidepressant effect [AGNOLI *et al.*, 1973] shown by trazodone. The action which the latter exerts on catecholamines occurs at higher doses than those found to affect serotonin.

It could, however, be possible that the inhibition of noradrenaline uptake may contribute to the antidepressant effect of trazodone. It is remarkable that, in contrast to tricyclic antidepressant agents, trazodone exerts only a minimal inhibition of noradrenaline uptake in the isolated atria of rats. This finding may be important in relation to the known cardiotoxicity shown by tricyclic antidepressant agents. The effect on brain dopamine is reminiscent of a stimulation of the dopaminergic system, a hypothesis in agreement with the toxic effect (vomiting) exerted by high doses of trazodone in dogs [RIVETT and SCORZA BARCELLONA, 1973].

Finally, it should be stressed that the neurochemical findings obtained with trazodone have been primarily obtained from studies on the whole brain, while a more careful analysis on discreet brain areas may be needed in order to detect possible specific interactions of trazodone with brain monoamines or aminoacids considered to be putative neurotransmitters.

References

AGNOLI, A.; PICCIONE, M.; CASACCHIA, M., and FAZIO, C.: Trazodone versus desipramine. A double-blind study on the rapidity of the antidepressive effect. Mod. Probl. Paediat., vol. 9, pp. 189–197 (Karger, Basel 1974).

AMIN, M.; BAN, T. A., and KLINGNER, A.: Trazodone in the treatment of affective disorders. Curr. ther. Res. *15:* 781–788 (1973).

ANGELUCCI, L.: Considerations on biochemical studies with trazodone. Mod. Probl. Paediat., vol. 9, pp. 65–75 (Karger, Basel 1974).

ANTONELLI, F.; DE GREGORIO, M., and DIONISIO, A.: Trazodone in the treatment of psychoneuroses: a double-blind study. Curr. ther. Res. *15:* 799–804 (1973).

BAIOCCHI, L.; CHIARI, A.; FRIGERIO, A., and RIDOLFI, P.: Analytical profile of trazodone. Arzneimittelforsch. *23:* 400–406 (1973 a).

BAIOCCHI, L.; CHIARI, A.; FRIGERIO, A., and RIDOLFI, P.: Personal commun. (1973 b).

BAN, T. A.; AMIN, M.; NAIR, N. P. V., and ENGELSMAN, F.: Comprehensive clinical studies with trazodone in Canada. Mod. Probl. Paediat., vol. 9, pp. 110–126 (Karger, Basel 1974).

BAN, T. A. and LEHMANN, H. E.: Systematic clinical studies with trazodone: methodological aspects. Curr. ther. Res. *15:* 764–768 (1973).

BERGMEYER, U. H.; BERNT, E.; MÖLLERING, H. und PFLEIDER, G.: In BERGMEYER Methoden der Enzymatischen Analyse: 2nd ed., p. 1651 (Verlag Chemie, Weinheim/B 1970).

BERNT, E. and BERGMEYER, H. U.: In BERGMEYER Methoden der Enzymatischen Analyse; 2nd ed., p. 1659 (Verlag Chemie, Weinheim/B 1970).

CARLSSON, A.; CORRODI, H.; FUXE, K., and HÖKFELT, T.: Effect of antidepressant drugs on the depletion of intraneuronal brain 5-hydroxytryptamine stores caused by 4-menthyl-α-ethyl-meta-tyramine. Europ. J. Pharmacol. *5:* 357–366 (1969).

CASSANO, G. B.; CASTROGIOVANNI, P., and CONTI, L.: Clinical evaluation of Trazodone in the treatment of depression. Mod. Probl. Paediat., vol. 9, pp. 198–203 (Karger, Basel 1974).

CATANESE, B. and LISCIANI, R.: Investigations on the absorption and distribution of trazodone or AF 1161 in rats, dogs and humans. Boll. chim. farm. *109:* 369 –373 (1970).

CHANG, C. C.: A sensitive method for spectrophotofluorometric assay of catecholamines. Int. J. Neuropharmacol. *3:* 643–649 (1964).

CONSOLO, S.; LADINSKY, H.; PERI, G., and GARATTINI, S.: Effect of central stimulant and depressants on mouse brain acetylcholine and choline levels. Europ. J. Pharmacol. *18:* 251–255 (1972).

DA PRADA, M. and PLETSCHER, A.: Acceleration of the cerebral dopamine turnover by chlorpromazine. Experientia *22:* 465–466 (1966).

DE GREGORIO, M. and DIONISIO, A.: A controlled clinical study of a new antidepressant (trazodone). Panminerva med. *13:* 27–30 (1971).

FUJITA, T.; YAMATO, C.; TAKAHASHI, T., and OHTAKE, S.: Absorption, tissue distribution, excretion and metabolism of ^{14}C-labelled trazodone hydrochloride in rats and rabbits. Mod. Probl. Paediat., vol. 9, pp. 56–64 (Karger, Basel 1974).

GARATTINI, S.: Effect of amphetamine and fenfluramine on monoamines. Vie méd. Canad. franç. *2:* 318–324 (1973).

GARATTINI, S.; FANELLI, R.; JORI, A.; CONSOLO, S.; LADINSKY, H., and SAMANIN, R.: Pharmacological and biochemical on piribedil (ET 495). Proc. Int. Symp. Trivastal, Monastir. (in press, 1972).

GHEZZI, D.; SAMANIN, R.; BERNASCONI, S.; TOGNONI, G.; GERNA, M., and GARATTINI, S.: Effects of tymoleptics on fenfluramine-induced depletion of brain serotonin in rats. Europ. J. Pharmacol. *24:* 205–210 (1973).

GIACALONE, E. and VALZELLI, L.: A spectrofluorometric method for the simultaneous determination of 2-(5-hydroxyindol-3-yl) ethylamine (serotonin) and 5-hydroxyindol-3-yl-acetic acid in the brain. Pharmacology *2:* 171–175 (1969).

HÄGGENDAL, J.: An improved method for fluorimetric determination of small amounts of adrenaline and noradrenaline in plasma and tissues. Acta physiol. scand. *59:* 242–254 (1963).

KANEKO, T. and YAMATSU, K.: Personal commun. (1972).

KNOBEL, M.: Trazodone and psychosomatic medicine. Curr. ther. Res. *15:* 789–798 (1973).

KORF, J.; OTTEMA, S., and VAN DER VEEN, I.: Fluorimetric determination of homovanillic acid in biological material after isolation on sephadex G-10. Analyt. Biochem. *40:* 187–191 (1971).

LONGO, V. G. and SCOTTI DE CAROLIS, A.: Pharmacological features of trazodone. Mod. Probl. Paediat., vol. 9, pp. 4–10 (Karger, Basel 1974).

MEEK, J. L. and NEFF, N. H.: The rate of formation of 3-methoxy-4-hydroxyphenylethyleneglycol sulfate in brain as an estimate of the rate of formation of norepinephrine. J. Pharmacol. exp. Ther. *184:* 570–575 (1973).

NAHORSKI, S. R.: Fluorometric measurement of glutamine and asparagine using enzymic methods. Analyt. Biochem. *42:* 136–142 (1971).

NAIR, N. P. V.; BAN, T. A.; HONTELA, S., and CLARKE, R.: Trazodone in the treatment of organic brain syndromes with special reference to psychogeriatrics. Curr. ther. Res. *15:* 769–775 (1973).

PALAZZO, G.: Chemistry of trazodone. Curr. ther. Res. *15:* 745–748 (1973).

RIVETT, K. F. and SCORZA BARCELLONA, P.: Toxicology of trazodone. Mod. Probl. Paediat., vol. 9, pp. 76–86 (Karger, Basel 1974).

SAELENS, J. K.; ALLEN, M. P., and SIMKE, J. P.: Determination of acetylcholine and choline by an enzymatic assay. Arch. int. Pharmacodyn. *186:* 279–286 (1970).

SCHANBERG, S. M.; SCHILDKRAUT, J. J.; BREESE, G. R., and KOPIN, I. J.: Metabolism of normetanephrine-H^3 in rat brain. Identification of conjugated 3-methoxy-4-hydroxphenylglycol as the major metabolite. Biochem. Pharmacol. *17:* 247–254 (1968).

SILVESTRINI, B.; CIOLI, V.; BURBERI, S., and CATANESE, B.: Pharmacological properties of AF 1161, a new psychotropic drug. Int. J. Neuropharmacol. *7:* 587–599 (1968).

SILVESTRINI, B. and LISCIANI, R.: Pharmacology of trazodone. Curr. ther. Res. *15:* 749–754 (1973).

SILVESTRINI, B. and QUADRI, E.: Investigations on the specificity of the so-called analgesic activity of non-narcotic drugs. Europ. J. Pharmacol. *12:* 231–235 (1970).

TAYLOR, K. M. and LAVERTY, R.: The effect of chlordiazepoxide, diazepam and nitrazepam on catecholamine metabolism in regions of the rat brain. Europ. J. Pharmacol. *8:* 296–301 (1969).

TOZER, T. N.; NEFF, N. H., and BRODIE, B. B.: Application of steady state kinetics to the synthesis rate and turnover time of serotonin in the brain of normal and reserpine-treated rats. J. Pharmacol. exp. Ther. *153:* 177–182 (1966).

UCHA UDABE, R.: Clinical experience with a new psychotropic drug, trazodone. Curr. ther. Res. *15:* 755–763 (1973).

YAMATO, C.; TAKAHASHI, T., and FUJITA, T.: Studies on metabolism of trazodone metabolic fate of (^{14}C) trazodone hydrochloride in rats. Xenobiotica (in press, 1973).

YAMATSU, K.; KANEKO, T.; YAMANISHI, Y.; KITAHARA, A., and OHTAKE, S.: A possible mechanism of central action of trazodone in rats. Mod. Probl. Paediat., vol. 9, 11–17 (Karger, Basel 1974).

Author's address: Prof. SILVIO GARATTINI, Istituto di Ricerche Farmacologiche Mario Negri, Via Eritrea 62, *I-20157 Milano* (Italy)

Trazodone. Mod. Probl. Pharmacopsychiat., vol. 9, pp. 47–51,
ed. Th. A. Ban, Montreal, Que., and B. Silvestrini, Rome (Karger, Basel 1974)

Effects of Trimeprazine, Trimeprimine and Trazodone on Conditioned Behaviour of Rats Using a Method of Discriminated Continuous Avoidance

Gian Luigi Gatti

Istituto Superior di Sanità, Roma

Previous investigations have shown that by using the discriminated continuous avoidance method (lever pressing avoidance, Sidman type) modified by Gatti and Bovet [1963], it is possible to observe not only quantitative but also qualitative differences among various psychotropic drugs.

In the last few years this methodology was employed in the study of over 50 substances including many phenothiazine, butyrophenone, benzodiazepine and iminodibenzyl derivatives. The first results, concerning some phenothiazine and butyrophenone derivatives, were published in a previous report [Gatti, 1967]. This paper reports the results obtained with trimeprazine, trimeprimine, and trazodone.

Materials and Methods

The modified discriminated continuous lever pressing avoidance technique (Sidman) was used in male Wistar rats. Shocks of 1.5 mA and 2-sec duration were given at intervals of 30 sec, with the light turning on, if the rats did not press the lever. Each response turned off the light and started a response-shock interval of 30 sec. This consists of a first, dark phase of 18 sec, followed by a second phase of 12 sec during which the light goes on as a warning stimulus. Shocks can be avoided either by responding during the first (dark) phase of the response-shock interval, or by responding during the second (lighted) phase of the response-shock interval, therefore turning off the light and avoiding the shock. In control conditions most animals progressively suppress the responses during the first phase of the response-shock interval, and eventually behave as in an instrumental avoidance situation (i. e. they give one response after each presentation of the warning stimulus).

Table I. Activity of different drugs on discriminated continuous lever-pressing avoidance in rats

Drug No.	Drug	ED_{40-50}, mg/kg s. c.
1	chlorpromazine	1.00
2	haloperidol	0.10
3	fluphenazine	0.1
4	trazodone	100.00
5	trimeprimine	100.00
6	trimeprazine	50.00

However, this cannot be considered as an instrumental avoidance test: responses given prior to the appearance of the warning stimulus (which can reappear in large numbers after certain drug treatments) do not have the neutral effect of intertrial responses, but start an entirely new cycle as in continuous avoidance test.

Furthermore, the dose was established for each drug which reduces by 40–50 % an arbitrary index (defined as operative response: OR). The OR is the ratio between the sum of the conditioned responses (CR), unconditioned responses (UR) and anticipatory responses (AR), and the sum of the conditioned stimuli (CS) and unconditioned stimuli (US) received. This ratio may be expressed as follows:

$$OR = \frac{CR + UR + AR}{CS + US}$$

Results

The approximate ED_{40-50} of 6 drugs are shown in table I. Results obtained with chlorpromazine (1), haloperidol (2) and fluphenazine (3) belong to the experiments already reported [GATTI, 1967]. Nevertheless, they are being included in this section for comparison.

Figure 1 illustrates the composition of OR at the time of its reduction by 40–50 %. The 6 drugs included in table I have been compared using two different criteria: comparison between the responses and comparison between the drugs.

At a dose of 100 mg/kg s. c. trazodone (4) decreases the OR by 45 %. CR represents 55 % of the total number of responses, UR 20 % and AR 25 %. No biphasic effect was observed from the dose of 5 mg/kg (OR decreased by 3 %) up to the dose of 100 mg/kg.

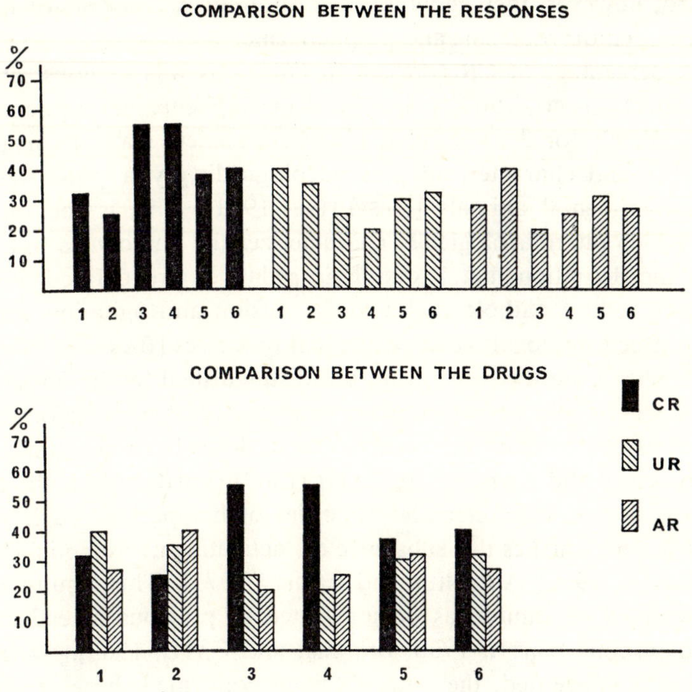

Fig. 1

At a dose of 100 mg/kg s. c. trimeprimine (5) decreases the OR by 50 %. CR represents 38 % of the total number of responses, UR 30 % and AR 32 %. No biphasic effect was observed from the dose of 5 mg/kg (OR decreased by 5 %) up to the dose of 100 mg/kg.

At a dose of 50 mg/kg s. c. trimeprazine (6) decreases the OR by 40 %. CR represents 40 % of the total number of responses, UR 32 % and AR 28 %. A strict dose/effect relationship was observed without a biphasic effect starting from the dose of 1 mg/kg (decrease of OR equal to 5 %) up to the dose of 50 mg/kg.

Discussions and Conclusions

The results show that trazodone, trimeprimine and trimeprazine have the characteristics of neuroleptics as far as the loss of conditioned behaviour is concerned; however, they show marked differences from major neuroleptics, such as chlorpromazine and perphenazine.

A high percentage of CR (present in OR) – as was demonstrated in previous papers [GATTI, 1967] – is typical of fluphenazine, a phenothiazine used clinically for the treatment of certain anxiety states [STILLE and WHITE, 1971] and characterized pharmacologically by a poor sedative action in experimental animals [HESELTINE, 1961]. This is the type of behaviour which pharmacologically characterizes the anxiolytics in agreement with the definition that, 'Anxiolytic sedatives are defined as substances which reduce pathological anxiety, tension and agitation without therapeutic effects on cognitive or perceptual processes [BAN, 1971]'.

Like fluphenazine the three drugs are distinguished by the absence of a biphasic effect in their action, contrary to what occurs with major neuroleptics, such as chlorpromazine, which in small doses has mild stimulating effects [GONZALES and ROSS, 1961; GATTI, 1967]. Furthermore, the three drugs possess certain characteristic properties of haloperidol, such as increase of AR which makes this substance an 'activating neuroleptic' [JANSSEN, 1962; BAN, 1969; AHLENIUS and ENGEL, 1971]. This results in an improved control of stimuli, as demonstrated in previous investigations in rats and pigeons [GATTI, 1966; BIGNAMI and GATTI, 1969]. As far as trimeprimine is concerned, the data obtained confirmed those of JULOU *et al.* [1961].

On the basis of these data, it can be concluded that all the three drugs possess pharmacodynamic actions which classify them among the anxiolytics. Trazodone has a marked predominance of CR and an almost equivalent percentage of UR and AR; therefore, it appears the drug of choice for conflict situations such as those occurring in discriminated continuous avoidance conditioning.

References

AHLENIUS, S. and ENGEL, J.: Effects of small doses of haloperidol on timing behaviour. J. Pharm. Pharmacol. *23:* 301–302 (1971).

BAN, T. A.: Psychopharmacology (Williams & Wilkins, Baltimore 1969).

BAN, T. A.: Methodological problems in the clinical evaluation of anxiolytic drugs; in VINAR, VOTAVA and BRADLEY Advances in neuropsychopharmacology (North Holland, Amsterdam 1971).

BIGNAMI, G. and GATTI, G. L.: Analysis of drugs effects on multiple fixed ratio 33. Fixed interval 5 min in pigeons. Psychopharmacologia, Berl. *15:* 310–332 (1969).

GATTI, G. L.: Comparative conditioning studies of drugs in laboratory animals; in BULL, COLE, DENIKER, HIPPIUS and BRADLEY Neuropsychopharmacology (Excerpta Medica Foundation, Amsterdam 1967).

GATTI, G. L. and BOVET, D.: Pharmacology of instrumental avoidance conditioning; in VOTAVA, HORVATH and VINAR Psychopharmacological methods (Pergamon Press, Oxford 1963).

GONZALES, R. C. and ROSS, S.: The effects of chlorpromazine on the cause of discrimination reversal learning. J. comp. physiol. Psychol. *54:* 645–681 (1961).

HESELTINE, W.: Pharmacological properties of fluphenazine; in Fluphenazine in anxiety and tension (Birchall, Liverpool 1961).

JANSSEN, P.: Pharmacologie comparée de l'halopéridol et du triperidol. Encephale *51:* 582–601 (1962).

STILLE, G. and WHITE, T.: Correlation between pharmacology and clinic; in VINAR, VOTAVA and BRADLEY Advances in neuropsychopharmacology (North Holland, Amsterdam 1971).

JULOU, *et al.:* Proprietés pharmacodynamiques générales du (diméthylamino-3-methyl-2-propyl-1)-5-iminodibenzyle (7. 162 R. P.) et de ses isomères optiques, droit (10. 633 R. P.) et gauche (10. 645 R. P.). C. R. Soc. Biol *155:* 307–312 (1961).

Author's address: Prof. G. GATTI, Istituto Superior di Sanità, Viale Regina Elena 299, *I-00181 Roma* (Italy)

Trazodone. Mod. Probl. Pharmacopsychiat., vol. 9, pp. 52–55,
ed. Th. A. Ban, Montreal, Que., and B. Silvestrini, Rome (Karger, Basel 1974)

Discussion on Pharmacological Features of Trazodone

E. F. DOMINO
Department of Pharmacology, University of Michigan, Ann Arbor

A review of the animal pharmacology of trazodone leaves one with a frustrated feeling. It is not easy to classify this drug as a classic antianxiety, antidepressant or neuroleptic agent on the basis of conventional animal tests.

First of all, is there a pharmacology of trazodone? The answer, of course, is a resounding yes! In fact, there is too much pharmacology [SILVESTRINI *et al.*, 1968]. Trazodone is a sedative with a wide spectrum of actions. It may be of help for us to update the comparative pharmacological profile of trazodone with other classes of central nervous system depressants. The actions of the antianxiety benzodiazepines, the neuroleptic phenothiazines and antidepressant tricyclics are compared to trazodone in table I. All four classes of drugs cause sedation and EEG synchronization but with widely different dose-effect and time-action curves. Especially important to note is that the benzodiazepines and trazodone also cause, in low dosage, EEG fast activity in man. However, they differ in their actions on the sleep cycle. Trazodone depresses REM sleep while benzodiazepines depress stages III and IV sleep. KANEKO *et al.* [1973] have pointed out that the effects of trazodone on REM sleep differ from those of imipramine. Trazodone had no antireserpine activity in a dose which suppressed REM sleep while imipramine suppressed REM sleep in a dose which also antagonized reserpine.

The four classes of drugs can also be distinguished on the basis of their effects on self-stimulation behavior. The benzodiazepines facilitate, the neuroleptics and trazodone depress, while the tricyclics have no significant effect or depress slightly self-stimulation. The four classes of drugs are also readily distinguished by their interactions with the amphetamines. The

Table I. Comparative pharmacological profile of trazodone with other psychotropic drugs

Action or test	Antianxiety benzo-diazepines	Neuroleptic pheno-thiazines	Anti-depressant tricyclics	Trazo-done
Sedation	+	+	+	+
EEG				
Slow waves	+	+	+	+
Fast waves (man)	+	0	0	+
Sleep				
Stage REM	0	0	–	–
Stages III and IV	– –	0 to +	0 to +	0
Reserpine antagonism	0	–	+	0
Self-stimulation	+++	–	0 to –	0 to –
Amphetamine antagonism	0	+++	– –	+
Dopa potentiation	0	– –	++	0 to –
α-Adrenergic antagonist	0	++	– –	+
Cholinergic antagonist	0	0 to ++	0 to ++	0
5-HTP potentiation	0	0	0	+
Brain				
5-HT	0	0	0	+
5-HIAA	0	+	0	–
5-HT antagonism				
Bronchospasm	0	+	0	++
Rabbit stomach	0	+	0	++

0 = No effect; + = enhanced; – = reduced.

benzodiazepines have no significant effect. Neuroleptics and trazodone reduce, while tricyclics potentiate amphetamine actions.

In view of the fact that amphetamines act on the adrenergic system, it is of interest to examine the effects of these four classes of psychotropic drugs for α-adrenergic blockade. While benzodiazepines have no significant adrenergic blocking actions, the tricyclic antidepressants potentiate adrenergic agonists and neuroleptics are α-adrenergic antagonists. Interestingly, trazodone is an α-adrenergic antagonist peripherally. Centrally, it slightly antagonizes dopa in contrast to the marked effects of the neuroleptics. Tricyclics significantly potentiate dopa while the benzodiazepines have no particular effect.

Trazodone has no anticholinergic effects while neuroleptics and tricyclic antidepressants are anticholinergic. The actions of trazodone on the serotonergic (5-HT) system are most complex. Prof. LONGO has just reported to us that on the 5-HTP test trazodone potentiates the induced tremor and splayed hind legs. This is an effect similar to what one would expect with drugs like chlorimipramine which selectively block 5-HT uptake in contrast to most tricyclic antidepressants which block catecholamine uptake. Strangely, trazodone also increases 5-HT and decreases 5-HIAA brain levels similar to an MAO inhibitor, which it is not. These findings are compatible with a central 5-HT agonist action. Yet peripherally trazodone shows a rather remarkable and highly selective antagonism of 5-HT bronchospasm and contraction of rabbit stomach. In view of its demonstrated central actions, it would be extremely important to test the effects of trazodone on 5-HT suppression in the lateral geniculate nucleus or the firing rate of 5-HT-containing neurons in raphé nucleus.

To summarize – what conclusions can we draw? It is obvious that we are dealing with a chemical that has a very complex pharmacology. Clearly it is not a placebo, but a chemical that cannot be easily classified except that it is a sedative with a different animal pharmacological spectrum. If it were your decision alone, would you have trazodone tested in man as a possible psychotropic drug? I am sure most of you would agree with the decision of our colleagues at Angelini Francesco to proceed with human trials to determine if trazodone has indeed a place in clinical therapy. I believe we are fortunate to be able to hear our colleagues from many different countries discuss their clinical experiences with this complicated drug. Certainly, from the point of view of its animal pharmacology trazodone would be a most interesting agent to investigate clinically as an anti-anxiety, antidepressant and soporific drug. As many of you know, our Italian and Japanese colleagues have had some interesting clinical experiences with this drug. In addition, BAN *et al.* [1973] in Montreal have reported some therapeutic benefit with this drug. It remains for future research, both basic and clinical, to fully assess the place of trazodone in our psychotropic armamentarium.

References

BAN, T. A.; LEHMANN, H. E.; AMIN, M.; GALVAN, L.; NAIR, N. P. V.; VERGARA, L., and ZOCH, C.: Comprehensive clinical studies with trazodone. Current therap. Res. *15:* 540–551 (1973).

KANEKO, T.; YAMATSU, K., and OHTAKE, S.: Effects of trazodone on sleep-wakefulness cycle of rats. Jap. J. Pharmacol. suppl. *23:* 81–132 (1973).

SILVESTRINI, B.; CIOLI, V.; BURBERI, S., and CATANESE, B.: Pharmacological properties of AF1161, a new psychotropic drug. Int. J. Neuropharmacol. *7:* 587–599 (1968).

Author's address: Prof. E. F. DOMINO, MD, Department of Pharmacology, University of Michigan, *Ann Arbor, MI 48104* (USA)

Trazodone. Mod. Probl. Pharmacopsychiat., vol. 9, pp. 56–64,
ed. Th. A. Ban, Montreal, Que., and B. Silvestrini, Rome (Karger, Basel 1974)

Absorption, Tissue Distribution, Excretion and Metabolism of ^{14}C-Labelled Trazodone Hydrochloride in Rats and Rabbits

T. FUJITA, C. YAMATO, T. TAKAHASHI and S. OHTAKE

Department of Drug Metabolism, Section of Experimental Research Therapeutics, Research and Development Division, Eisai Co., Ltd.

Introduction

The absorption, excretion and tissue distribution of trazodone (abbreviated as TR) hydrochloride administered orally or intravenously in rats, dogs and humans have been determined using the spectrofluorimetric method of CATANESE and LISCIANI [1970].

This paper reports a detailed investigation on absorption, tissue distribution, excretion and metabolites of TR in rats and rabbits using ^{14}C-labelled trazodone (abbreviated as [^{14}C]TR) hydrochloride.

Methods

[^{14}C] TR hydrochloride synthetized as outlined in figure 1 had a specific radioactivity of 27.3 μCi/mg and was confirmed to be pure on the thin-layer chromatograms.

Male Wistar rats weighing 150–220 g and male albino rabbits weighing 1.8–2.2 kg were maintained on a pellet diet supplied by Nihon Crea Co., Ltd. Animals were fasted for 18–20 h but tap water was available *ad libitum*. Animals were given an aqueous solution (1 ml/100 g body weight) of [^{14}C] TR hydrochloride orally at single dosages of 4 or 20 mg/kg. Radioactivities in blood, tissue and feces were determined by a liquid scintillation counter (Aloka model LSC-601) following the combustion using a Tri-Carb Sample Oxidizer (model 305) (fig. 2).

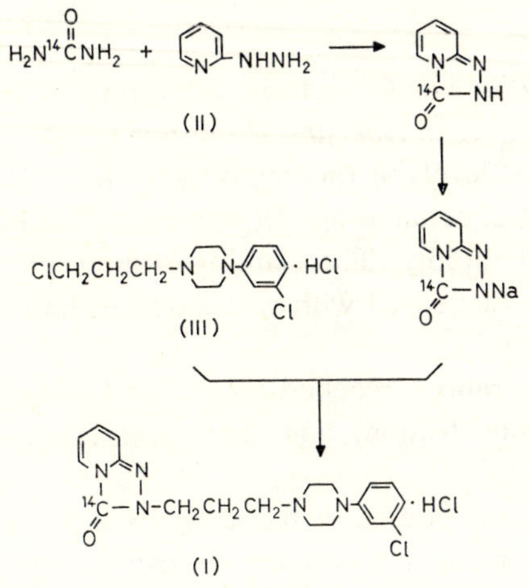

Fig. 1. Synthesis of [^{14}C]TR hydrochloride.

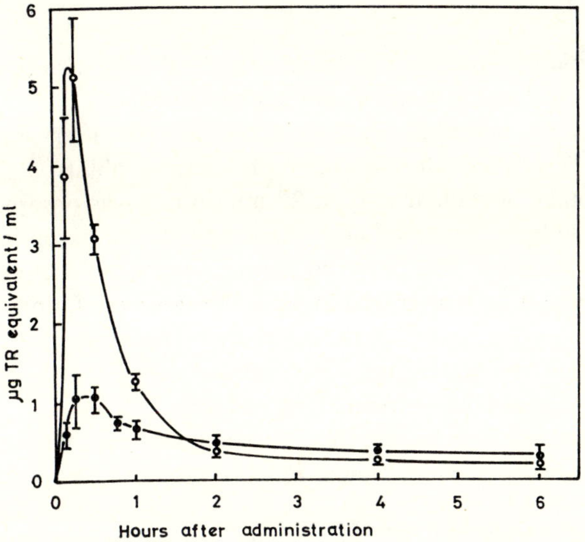

Fig. 2. Blood levels of radioactivity after oral administration of [^{14}C]-TR (20 mg/kg) in the rat fasted for 18–20 h (○) and in the nonfasted rat (●). Values represent means ±SE of three experiments.

Results and Discussion

Blood Level of Radioactivity following Oral Administration of [^{14}C]TR Hydrochloride 4 mg/kg in Rats and Rabbits

As shown in figure 3, the blood levels of radioactivity in rats attained already a maximum of 0.63 μg TR equivalent/ml 15 min after oral ingestion, and was thereafter decreased rapidly. The semilogarithmic plotting showed that the blood level in rats decreased with two different half-lives of 19.3 min and 5.9 h, respectively.

In contrast, the blood levels in rabbits reached a peak of 1.08 μg TR equivalent/ml 3 h after oral administration, and then declined slowly (fig. 4).

The discrepancy between the time course of blood levels in rats and that in rabbits might mainly come from a difference in gastric emptying time of both animals. This suggestion seems to be supported by the following: maximum blood level of 5.1 μg TR equivalent/ml was observed 15 min after oral administration of [^{14}C]TR hydrochloride 20 mg/kg in the rat fasted for 20 h, while the blood level following oral ingestion in the non-fasted rat attained a peak of 1.0 μg TR equivalent/ml at 30 min and thereafter declined slowly.

Tissue Distribution of Radioactivity Following Oral Administration of [^{14}C]TR Hydrochloride 4 mg/kg in Rats and Rabbits

Figure 5 shows the tissue distribution of radioactivity after oral administration of [^{14}C]TR hydrochloride 4 mg/kg in rats and rabbits.

The highest uptake of radioactivity at 20 min in rats was observed in liver, followed by kidney, pancreas and adrenal, with the exception of small intestine and stomach. The tissue concentrations of radioactivity in brain at 20 min, 6 h and 24 h after oral ingestion in rats were found to be 0.19, 0.01 and 0.006 μg TR equivalent/g wet tissue, respectively.

On the other hand, the highest uptake of radioactivity at 3 h in rabbits was noted in kidney, followed by adrenal, lung and liver.

The residual radioactivity in the tissues examined was almost not detectable 168 h following oral ingestion in rats and rabbits.

Urinary and Fecal Excretions of Radioactivity after Oral Administration of [^{14}C]TR Hydrochloride 4 mg/kg in Rats and Rabbits

As shown in figure 6, the total excretion of radioactivity in rats was 74.1 % of the dose within 24 h and 95.1 % during the first 7 days. Approxi-

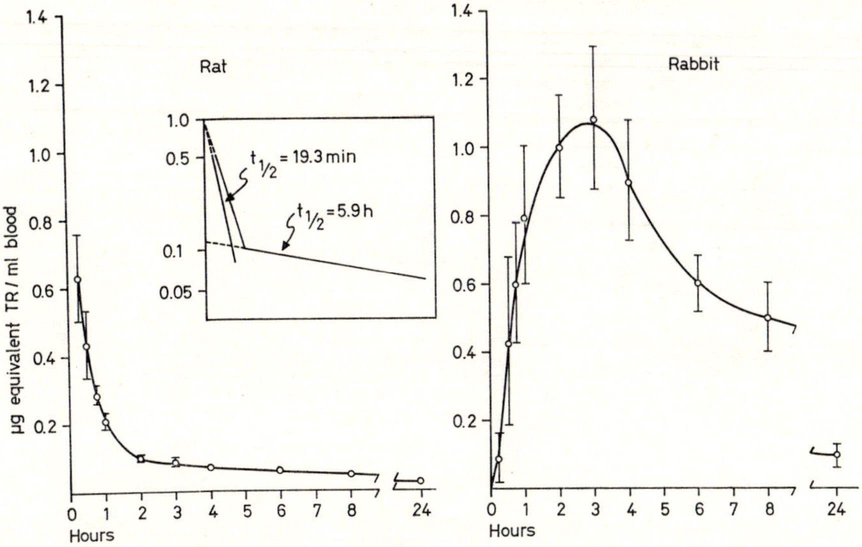

Fig. 3. Blood level of radioactivity after oral administration of [14C] TR hydrochloride, 4 mg/kg in rats (n = 4) and rabbits (n = 5). Data are expressed as means of µg trazodone equivalent/ml blood ± SE.

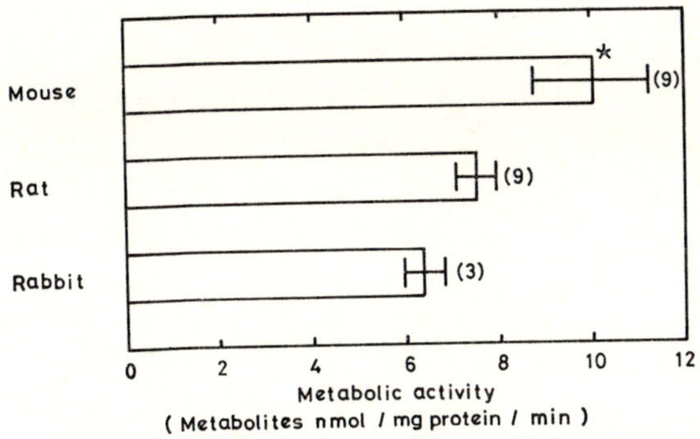

Fig. 4. Metabolic activity of [14C]TR in mouse, rat and rabbit liver microsomes. [14C]TR (0.8 µmol) was incubated with 2 ml of the mixture consisting of 1 ml microsomal suspension of each animal, 0.6 µmol NADP, 15 µmol G-6-P, 3.6 IU G-6-P dehydrogenase, 0.1 µmol EDTA, 30 µmol $MgCl_2$ and 0.1 M Tris-HCl buffer (pH 7.4) for 10 min. The number of animals in each group is shown in parentheses. * Significantly different from rat and rabbit liver microsomes ($p < 0.01$).

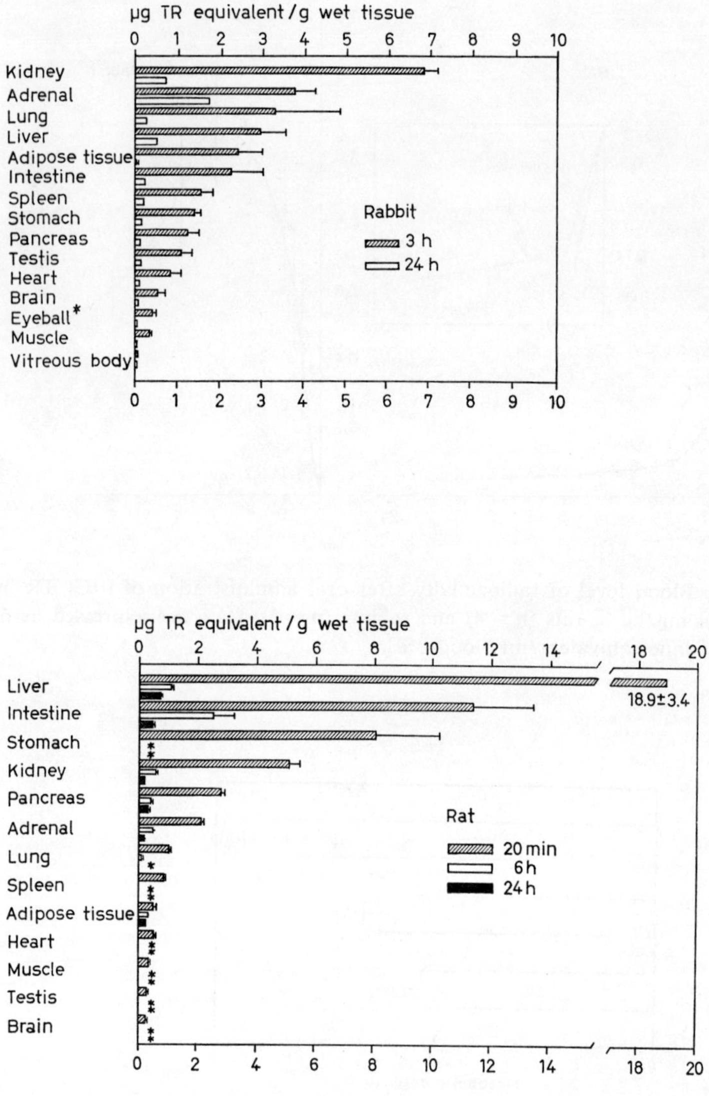

Fig. 5. Tissue distribution of radioactivity after oral administration of [^{14}C]TR hydrochloride 4 mg/kg in rats and rabbits. Data are expressed as means of µg trazodone equivalent/g wet tissue ± SE. Three animals were used in each experiment except for the 24-hour experiment in the rabbit (n = 2). * Eyeball excluding vitreous body.

mately equal amounts of the total radioactivity excreted were recognized in urine and feces during the first 7 days. In contrast, the urinary and fecal excretions of radioactivity in rabbits were 65.4 and 13.4 per cent of the dose within 24 h, and 67.8 and 20.8 per cent during the first 4 days, respectively.

The main route of elimination of [^{14}C]TR hydrochloride orally administered was fecal in rats and urinary in rabbits. These facts might be reflected in the result that the highest uptake of radioactivity was observed in the liver in rats and in the kidney in rabbits.

Biliary excretion of radioactivity after oral administration of [^{14}C]TR hydrochloride 4 mg/kg in rats was 50 % of the radioactivity dosed during the first hour and 80 % within 8 h. Accordingly, the occurrence of enterohepatic circulation of [^{14}C]TR orally administered in rats was suggested from these findings.

It is evident that [^{14}C]TR administered orally is absorbed very well from the gastrointestinal tract in both animals.

Urinary and Biliary Metabolites of
[^{14}C]TR Hydrochloride 4 mg/kg
Orally Administered in Rats and Rabbits

Two metabolites of TR were isolated from the urine of rats administered with [^{14}C]TR 4 mg/kg orally. One of these metabolites was identified as 2-{3- [4-(m-chloro-p-hydroxyphenyl)-1-piperazinyl]-propyl}-s-triazolo-[4,3a]-pyridin-3-(2H)-one (abbreviated as OH-TR, fig. 7) by thin layer chromatography, ultraviolet spectrophotometry, mass spectrometry and dilution analysis using the synthetic methoxy TR. The other metabolite was confirmed to be β-(3-oxo-s-triazolo-[4,3a]-pyridin-2-yl)-propionic acid (abbreviated as TPA, fig. 7) by the same methods using the synthetic TPA kindly supplied by Angelini Francesco ACRAF S.p.A.

The excretions of TR and its metabolites in the 24-hour urine and the 4-hour bile of rats and the 24-hour urine of rabbits are shown in table I, expressed as a percentage of the dose. The main metabolites in urine and bile of rats were unconjugated TPA and OH-TR glucuronide, respectively. In contrast, the main urinary excretes in rabbits were found to be OH-TR glucuronide and unconjugated TPA except for unknown polar metabolites. The urinary excretions of unchanged TR and unconjugated OH-TR were of low degree in both animals. The results reported by CATANESE and LISCIANI [1970] that a small amount of unchanged TR was excreted in the urine of the rat, was in agreement with our findings.

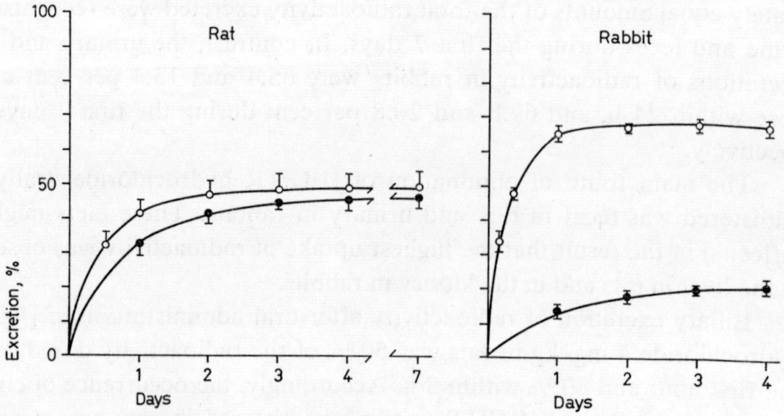

Fig. 6. Cumulative urinary and fecal excretions of radioactivity after oral administration of [^{14}C]TR hydrochloride 4 mg/kg in rats and rabbits. Data are expressed as a percentage of the dose ±SE. ○ = Urine; ● = feces.

Table I. Excretion percentages of trazodone and its metabolites in urine and bile after oral administration of [^{14}C]TR hydrochloride 4 mg/kg in rats and rabbits (data are expressed as a percentage of the dose)

Metabolites	Rat		Rabbit
	urine[1]	bile[2]	urine[1]
Unchanged TR	2.9	0.6	0.5
OH-TR	4.8	0.8	0.5
Unknown basic metabolite	0	0	3.1
TPA	14.2	1.9	5.0
Glucuronide of OH-TR	4.0	53.0	11.4
Glucuronide of TPA	3.6	0.5	2.2
Unknown polar metabolites	11.8	20.5	42.7
Total	41.3	77.3	65.4

1 0- to 24-hour urine.
2 0- to 4-hour bile.

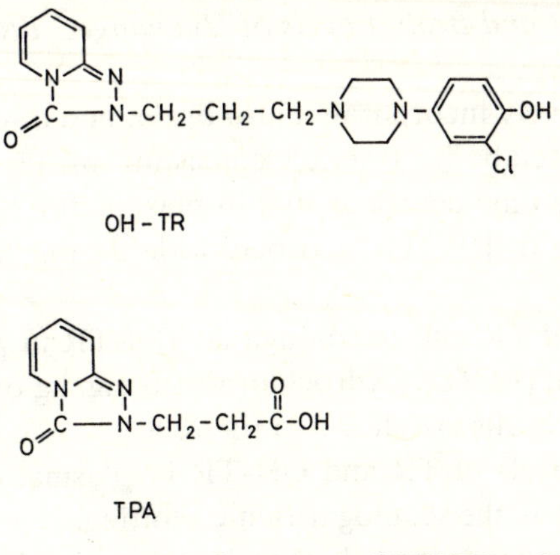

Fig. 7. Chemical structure of OH-TR and TPA.

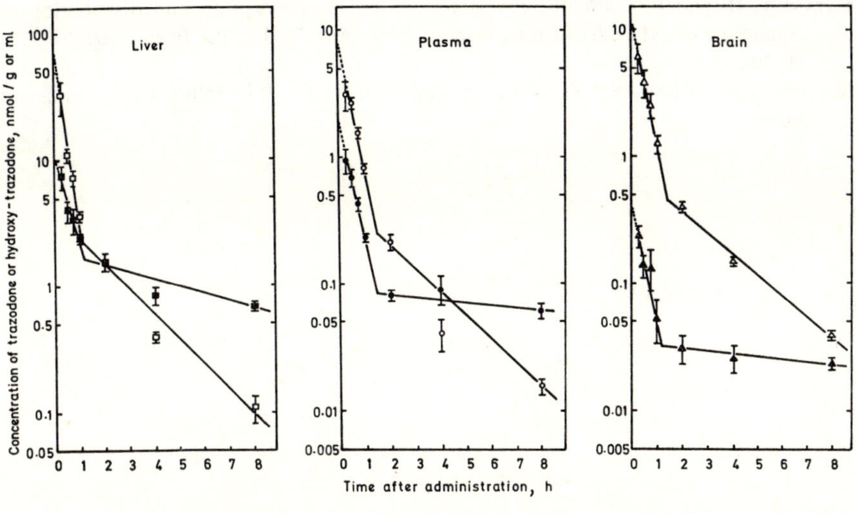

Fig. 8. Time course of liver, plasma and brain levels of unchanged TR and unconjugated OH-TR after oral administration of [14C]TR hydrochloride 20 mg/kg in rats. Data are expressed as means of three rats ± SE. Open symbols indicate unchanged TR, solid symbols indicate unconjugated OH-TR.

Time Course of Plasma, Liver and Brain Levels of Unchanged TR and OH-TR in Rats

TR and OH-TR were exclusively incorporated into brain, and also the radioactivity level of the basic metabolite fraction consisting of TR and OH-TR in brain showed the same time course as that in plasma during the first 8 h after oral administration of [^{14}C]TR hydrochloride 20 mg/kg in rats.

Thus, the levels of unchanged TR and unconjugated OH-TR in plasma, liver and brain of the rat given [^{14}C]TR hydrochloride 20 mg/kg orally were separately determined. The results are shown in figure 8.

All the time courses of the levels of TR and OH-TR in plasma, liver and brain were of the biphasic type in the semilogarithmic plotting.

The levels of TR in brain were significantly higher than those in plasma during the first 8 h after oral ingestion, while the levels of OH-TR in brain were apparently lower than those in plasma. These findings suggest that the affinity of TR to brain is higher than that to plasma.

References

CATANESE, B. and LISCIANI, R.: Investigations on the absorption and distribution of trazodone or AF 1161 in rats, dogs and humans. Boll. chim. farm. *109:* 369–373 (1970).

SUGIYAMA, K.; KONO, S.; YAMATO, C., and FUJITA, T.: J. Labelled Compounds (in press).

Author's address: Dr. T. FUJITA, Eisai Co. Ltd., Koishikawa 4, Bunkyo, *Tokyo* (Japan)

Trazodone. Mod. Probl. Pharmacopsychiat., vol. 9, pp. 65–75,
ed. Th. A. Ban, Montreal, Que., and B. Silvestrini, Rome (Karger, Basel 1974)

Considerations on Biochemical Studies with Trazodone

L. Angelucci and P. Bolle

Istituto di Farmacologia e Farmacognosia, University of Rome, Rome

As shown by Silvestrini *et al.* [1968, 1973], trazodone has a peculiar spectrum of pharmacological activity which leads one to consider this substance as a psychotropic drug characterized by such behavioral effects as calmness, reduced reactivity to distressing stimuli and reduction of the emotional component of the response to a painful stimulus.

It is of interest, therefore to establish whether the neuropsychopharmacological actions of trazodone are associated with changes in brain amine levels which are interfered with by neuroleptics, antidepressants and morphine-like analgesics.

Garattini [1969] has shown that trazodone can block the uptake of both serotonin and noradrenaline, and that some changes in the level of brain serotonin and noradrenaline may occur in the Sprague-Dawley rat, although inconsistently under the influence of this drug. Further, Garattini [1969] has found no variation in the turnover rate of noradrenaline in trazodone treated animals.

In this context, I would like to present some data obtained in our laboratory using the albino Swiss mouse and the Wistar rat. As shown in figure 1, trazodone if given by the intraperitoneal route, affects the concentrations of biogenic amines and 5-HIAA in the mouse brain. The quality and intensity of this effect is dose-related. In fact, with 5 mg/kg there is a decrease in the level of 5-HIAA and no significant variation in the level of the amines; with 25 mg/kg the decrease of 5-HIAA is accompanied by an increase in the level of 5-HT. With the highest dose used (50 mg/kg) there is a great variation in 5-HIAA and 5-HT levels but at the same time there is a decrease in brain NA and DA levels.

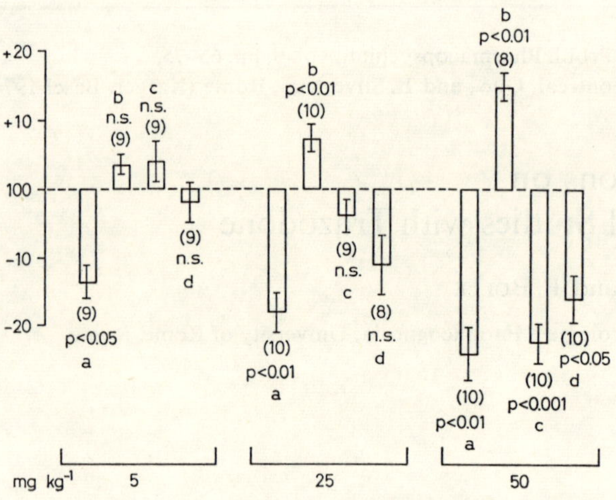

Fig. 1. Brain concentrations (percent of 8 controls ± SEM) of monoamines and 5-HIAA in the mouse following the i. p. injection of trazodone at different dose levels. The animals were sacrificed 1 h after the last of three doses given at 2-hour intervals. Difference versus saline 10 ml kg^{-1} controls (8). Number of animals in parentheses. Control values (ng g^{-1} ± SEM) were: 5-HIAA (*a* columns) 350 ± 17; 5-HT (*b* columns) 833 ± 12; NA (*c* columns) 326 ± 6; (*d* columns) 1,173 ± 51.

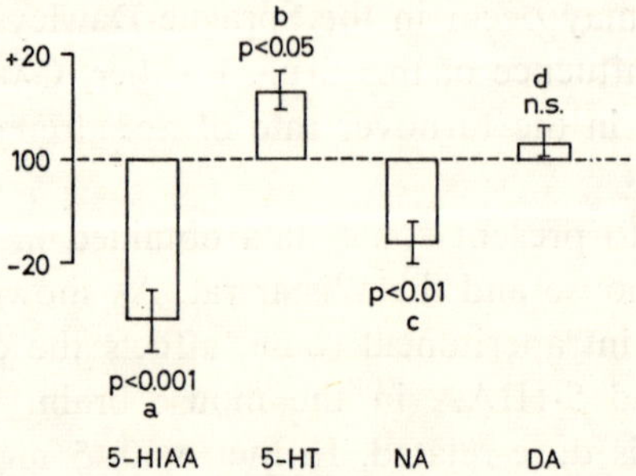

Fig. 2. Brain concentration (percent of controls ± SEM) of neuroamines and 5-HIAA in 8 rats following the i. p. injection of trazodone. The animals were sacrificed 1 h after the last of three 25 mg kg^{-1} doses given at 2-hour intervals. Difference versus saline 10 ml kg^{-1} controls (8). Control values (ng g^{-1} ± SEM) were: 5-HIAA 461 ± 20; 5-HT 745 ± 19; NA 422 ± 13; DA 941 ± 24.

We can conclude that in 'low' doses, trazodone has a selective action on brain 5-HT metabolism, while in 'high' doses the action is on catecholamine metabolism.

It should be noted that the behavioral effect of trazodone in animals receiving 'low' doses is a characteristic condition of quiesence with reduced motor activity. Reactivity to stimulation is reduced and there is an absence of any sign of catatonia and/or stereotypy. On the other hand, dosed beyond 50 mg/kg, the mouse becomes prostrated and clonic convulsions may appear.

In the rat (fig. 2), intraperitoneal injection of trazodone produces a similar picture with a decrease of 5-HIAA and an increase in 5-HT levels. However, an injection of 25 mg/kg results in a decrease of NA concentration.

Since in these experiments, monoamine and 5-HIAA levels were studied at a fixed time interval (1 h after treatment), the question arises whether the impact of the substance on catecholamines was a true function of the dose or the time pattern. As shown in figures 2 and 3, our studies seem to indicate the first alternative to be correct, i. e., a dose relationship. Figure 3 shows the concentration, at hourly intervals, of brain 5-HIAA and other monoamines in mice treated with a 'low' (15 mg/kg i. p.) dose of trazodone. The dose used is the ED_{50} for abolishing aggressiveness in isolated mice and is also the dose which consistently reduces conditioned avoidance reflexes. In the following 5 h there is a decrease of 5-HIAA level, associated with an increase in 5-HT concentration which is slow in comparison with the decrease of the acid metabolite and of shorter duration (3 h). In the same period no continuous variation of the levels NA and DA is observed, although a singular significant decrease in NA level is found at 15 min after the injection, and a parallel short-lived significant downshift for NA and DA levels is seen at 5 h.

In contrast to this picture, in mice treated with a 'high' dose of trazodone (60 mg/kg i. p.), the changes in 5-HIAA and 5-HT – which last longer than with the 'low' dose of 15 mg/kg – are associated with an early marked decline of the NA level which returns to normal in 90 min. The level of DA also shows an early short-lived significant decline. Again, at 5 h, NA and DA levels show a downshift, now with a longer duration in comparison with the 15 mg/kg dose (fig. 4).

The effects of trazodone on brain monoamine levels has also been studied by giving the drug to the mouse orally (fig. 5). There is an obvious early decline in 5-HIAA level, a delayed increase in 5-HT level, and an

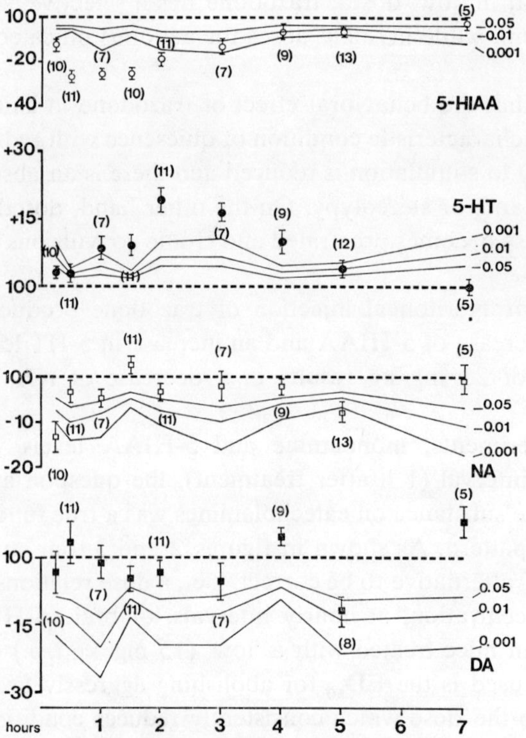

Fig. 3. Brain concentrations (each value is the mean in percent of 7–13 controls at each time, ± SEM; number of animals in parentheses) of monoamines and 5-HIAA in the mouse at differenct times from the i. p. injection of trazodone 15 mg kg^{-1}. Significance limits were obtained from 103 control animals. Total control values ($ng\ kg^{-1}$ ± SEM) were: 5-HIAA 375 ± 3; 5-HT 801 ± 4; NA 351 ± 3; DA 977 ± 4.

early, short-lived, fall in NA level at 1 h followed by a significant downshift at 5 h. The effect on 5-HT and 5-HIAA is still present at 9 h (fig. 5).

It is interesting to note that in animals treated twice a day for seven days the effect of trazodone on brain NA level is practically absent as compared with animals treated only once.

Except for changes in the NA level, these results are substantially in agreement with data obtained in the rat orally, and reported by YAMATSU *et al.* [1973]. It is possible that significant changes in NA and DA levels, as we found in rats and mice treated with trazodone, even at 'intermediate'

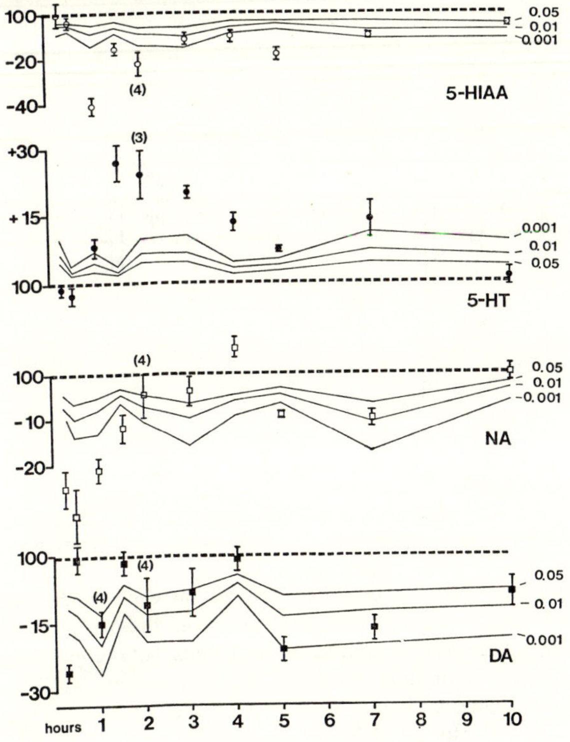

Fig. 4. Brain concentrations (each value is the mean in percent of 7–13 controls at each time, ±SEM from 5 animals, except as stated in parentheses) of monoamines and 5-HIAA in the mouse at different times after the i. p. injection of trazodone 60 mg kg^{-1}. Significance limits were obtained from 103 control animals. Total control values (ng g^{-1} ± SEM) were: 5-HIAA 375 ± 3; 5-HT 801 ± 4; NA 351 ± 3; DA 997 ± 4.

doses, were merely detected because of an accurate matching of 'treated' versus 'control' animals at each time and in each amine assay experiment.

The involvement of catecholamine level becomes the prominent feature of the brain biochemical variation induced by trazodone when a dose of 100 mg/kg i. p. is given to mice (fig. 6). As shown in figure 6, with 100 mg/kg i. p. (which produces prostration, impairment of motor reactivity and clonic convulsions), the fall in NA and DA levels equals about 60 and 75 % of normal, respectively (at 60 min); moreover, at this dose the action on the levels of 5-HT and its acid metabolite appears distorted in com-

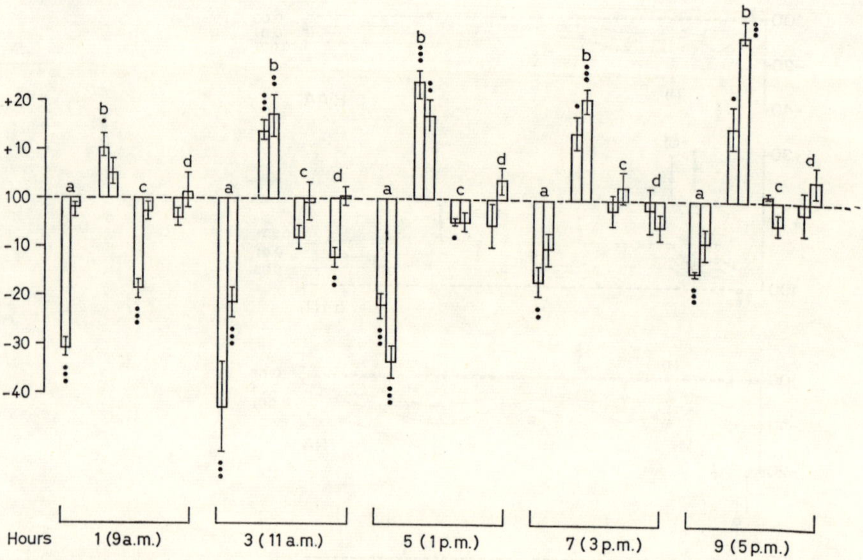

Fig. 5. Brain concentrations (percent of saline controls at each time, ±SEM) of monoamines and 5-HIAA in the mouse at different times from the o. s. administration of trazodone 100 mg kg^{-1}. Five treated animals at each time. Total control values (ng g^{-1} ±SEM) were: 5-HIAA (*a* columns) 374±4; 5-HT (*b* columns) 770±9; NA (c columns) 377±4; DA (d columns) 934±20 (n = 50). ·, ··, and ···: $p < 0.05$, $p < 0.01$, and $p < 0.001$, respectively. In each pair of columns: on the left, value in animals treated once only; on the right, value in animals treated twice a day (8 a. m. and 8 p. m.) for seven days.

parison with the action of 'low' doses. Indeed, there is now an early and short-lived fall of 5-HT levels, associated with the tendency to an increase in the 5-HIAA level; thereafter, the usual direction of changes in brain 5-HT and 5-HIAA is resumed with some irregularity (see 5-HT at 90 min). These peculiar aspects of the action of trazodone at 'high' doses in the mouse are confirmed by data obtained in rats injected intravenously with 35 mg/kg.

What can we learn from these data?

An answer to this question needs some preliminary considerations. The pharmacological actions of trazodone could be independent from a primary impingement of the drug on the regulatory function of central monoaminergic systems. The changes in the levels on monoamines might not be the basis of the response, but just an epiphenomenon. Against this inter-

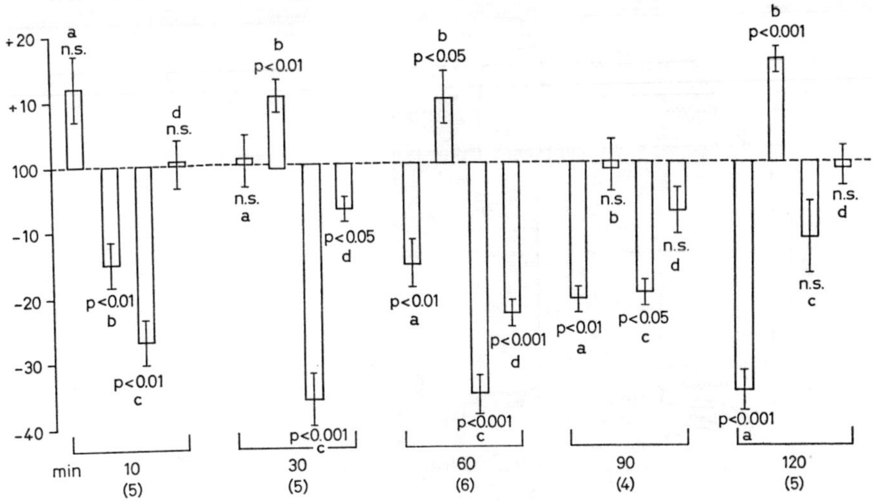

Fig. 6. Brain concentrations (percent of 6 saline controls at each time, ±SEM) of monoamines and 5-HIAA in the mouse at different times from the i. p. injection of trazodone 100 mg kg^{-1}. Zero time control values (ng g^{-1}±SEM) were: 5-HIAA (*a* columns) 368±12; 5-HT (*b* columns) 783±10; NA (*c* columns) 391±7; DA (*d* columns) 962±21. Number of animals in parentheses.

pretation is the parallelism of the time course of changes in the levels of 5-HT and its acid metabolite on the one hand, and on the other, the time course of the behavioral effects of trazodone, as well as of brain levels of unchanged trazodone [according to the data referred to by Fujita *et al.*, 1973]. At this symposium Fujita *et al.* [1973] have pointed out that the time course of the levels of unchanged trazodone in blood and brain of rats is biphasic, and that there are two different plasma half-lives: 19.3 min and 5.9 h, respectively. One wonders if the shorter one may coincide with the short-lived fall in NA levels, and the longer one with the long-lasting variations in levels of 5-HT and 5-HIAA, which are seen in the mouse with the highest doses of trazodone. This could place the focus onto the existence of a real relationship between the effects of trazodone on behavior and drug-induced variations in its central monoaminergic control.

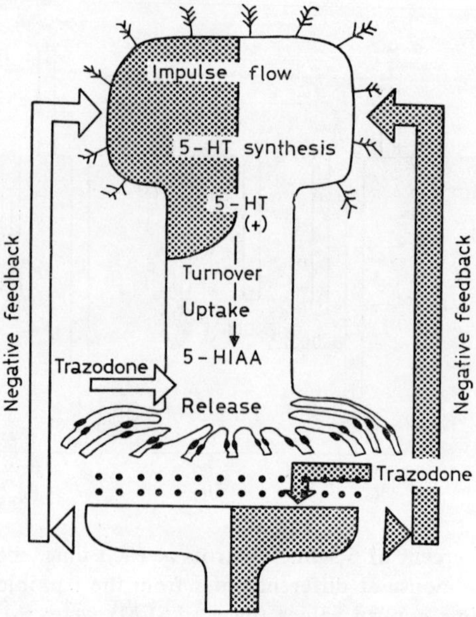

Fig. 7. A proposed schema for the action of trazodone on 5-HT metabolism. Hatched areas = activation, open areas = disactivation.

With regard to the meaning of variations in brain levels of monoamines in terms of functional variations of monoaminergic mechanism, the inconclusiveness of the former is obvious if turnover studies are not carried out, and if concentrations in discrete brain areas are not known.

However, we can reasonably assume that the increase in 5-HT and the decrease in 5-HIAA levels are consequent to a reduced turnover of the indolamine. Inhibition of MAO is ruled out by the concomitant decrease of NA levels obtained with high doses of trazodone. Moreover, GARATTINI [1969] has demonstrated that trazodone is devoid of any MAO inhibitor activity.

With regard to the fall in NA level induced by trazodone at higher doses, to argue whether we are dealing with an activation or disactivation of central noradrenergic circuits, would be futile not knowing how the turnover of NA is exactly affected by this drug.

However, GARATTINI [1973] has told us that he has found no variation in the level of MHPG.

Coming back to the turnover of brain 5-HT, it could be affected by

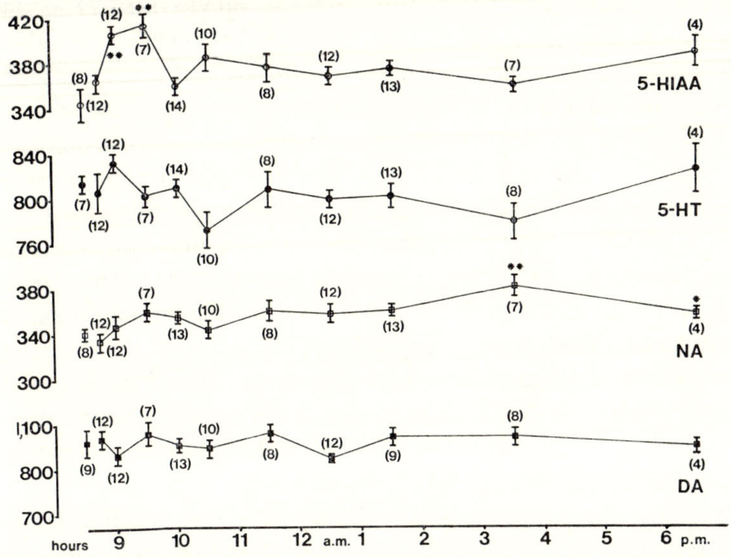

Fig. 8. Brain concentrations (ng g^{-1} ± SEM) of neuroamines in the mouse (light period) at different times from the i. p. injection of saline 10 ml kg^{-1}. The first value in each row is in normal animals, * and **, significant difference versus normal animals, with $p < 0.05$ and $p < 0.01$, respectively. Number of animals in parentheses.

trazodone in one, or both of two ways, as shown in figure 7. Firstly, the drug may directly inhibit the functional release of 5-HT. In this case the function of the serotoninergic neurone is reduced, even though the impulse flow can increase, and the typtaminergic receptor is less activated. This would lead to a decreased formation of 5-HIAA and to an increase in the 5-HT level from reduced utilization and stimulation of synthesis through a decreased negative feed-back mechanism starting post-synaptically.

Secondly, trazodone may stimulate the tryptaminergic receptor, and from this, through an increased negative feed-back mechanism, there follows a compensatory reduction of impulse flow, and of release and turnover of 5-HT, as well as a diminished production of 5-HIAA. The level of 5-HT may be higher than normal.

Both of these possibilities are compatible with some effects of trazodone *depending on the dose,* and taking into account the serotoninergic nature of the raphe nuclei, and the fact that here there are neurons which contain 5-HT and can be excited by 5-HT applied to their membranes

[BRAWLEY and DUFFIELD, 1972]. For instance, SILVESTRINI *et al.* [1968] have shown that a very low dose of trazodone, 0.5 mg/kg i. v., produces in the rabbit a synchronising effect and inhibits the arousal reaction (sedation, trophotropic action). On the other hand, YAMATSU *et al.* [1973] have shown in this symposium that trazodone at the high dose of 160 mg/kg p. o. reduces in the rat the amount of slow wave sleep and suppresses paradoxical sleep (ergotropic action, as with trycyclic antidepressants).

Even if SILVESTRINI *et al.* [1968] have shown that trazodone has a peripheral antiserotonin action, a central stimulating action on tryptaminergic receptors and a peripheral inhibiting action cannot be excluded.

ANDÉN *et al.* [1968] have given evidence for a central serotonin receptor stimulation by LSD, and have also shown that this drug at low doses reduces the turnover of 5-HT, and at high doses, accelerates the turnover of NA. Moreover, COSTA [1956] has found that LSD at low concentrations mimics the excitatory effects of 5-HT on rat uterus.

LSD evokes the opportunity of pointing out some peculiarities in the action of trazodone on brain amine levels. LSD at low doses slows down the turnover of 5-HT, producing an increase in brain 5-HT level and a decrease in brain 5-HIAA level [FREEDMAN, 1963]. At high doses LSD also reduces the levels of NA [FREEDMAN, 1963], and activates the ECoG [ELKES *et al.*, 1954].

In conclusion, the following points may be stressed:

1. The behavioural effect of trazodone appears strictly associated with drug-induced variations of brain monoamine levels and reduction of brain 5-HT turnover; both effect and variations appear dose-related.

2. Behavioral effects of trazodone need not be confined to a specific involvement of 5-HT or catecholamine; on the contrary, trazodone may affect the noradrenergic system (which in turn produces behavioral changes) by altering the central serotoninergic system.

3. The clinical usefulness of trazodone, or its role as an antidepressant, cannot be predicted only from brain biochemical changes induced in normal experimental animals. In fact, our knowledge of the relationship between brain monoamines and normal or disordered emotional activity is still limited.

These experiments have been conducted with the technical assistance of Mrs. ELDA VALLONE. Concentrations of 5-HIAA, 5-HT, NA and DA in the whole brain were estimated spectrofluorimetrically on the same tissue sample by the methods of MILLER *et al.* [1970] and WELCH and WELCH [1969] with some minor modifications.

References

ANDÉN, N. E.; CORRODI, H.; FUXE, K., and HÖKFELT, T.: Evidence for a central 5-hydroxytryptamine receptor stimulation by lysergic acid dietylamide. Brit. J. Pharmacol. *34:* 1–7 (1968).

BRAWLEY, P. and DUFFIELD, J. C.: The pharmacology of hallucinogens. Pharmacol. Rev. *24:* 31–66 (1972).

COSTA, E.: Effects of hallucinogenic and tranquilizing drugs on serotonin evoked uterine contractions. Proc. Soc. exp. Biol. Med. *91:* 39–41 (1956).

ELKES, J.; ELKES, C., and BRADLEY, P. B.: The effect of some drugs on the electrical activity of the brain and on behaviour. J. ment. Sci. *100:* 125–141 (1954).

FREEDMAN, D. X.: Psychotomimetic drugs and brain biogenic amines. Amer. J. Psychiat. *119:* 843–850 (1963).

FUJITA, T.; YAMATO, C.; TAKASAKI, T., and OHTAKE, S.: Absorption, tissue distribution, excretion and metabolism of ^{14}C-labelled trazodone hydrochloride in rats and rabbits. This Symposium (1973).

GARATTINI, S.: Personal commun. (1969).

GARATTINI, S.: Biochemical Studies with Trazodone, a new Psychoactive Drug. Mod. Probl. Paediat., vol. 9, pp. 29–46 (Karger, Basel 1974).

MILLER, F. P.; COX, R. H., jr.; SNODGRASS, W. R., and MAICKEL, R. P.: Comparative effects of *p*-chlorophenylalanine, *p*-chloroamphetamine and *p*-chloro-N-methylamphetamine on rat brain norepinephrine, serotonin and 5-hydroxyindole-3-acetic acid. Biochem. Pharmacol. *19:* 435–442 (1970).

SILVESTRINI, B.; CIOLI, V.; BURBERI, S., and CATANESE, B.: Pharmacological properties of AF 1161, a new psychotropic drug. Int. J. Neuropharmacol. *7:* 587–599 (1968).

SILVESTRINI, B. and LISCIANI, R.: Pharmacology of trazodone. Curr. Ther. Res. *20:* 754–799 (1963).

WELCH, A. S. and WELCH, B. L.: Solvent extraction method for simultaneous determination of norepinephrine, dopamine, serotonin, and 5-hydroxyindolacetic acid in a single mouse brain. Anal. Biochem. *30:* 161–179 (1969).

YAMATSU, K.; KANEKO, T.; YAMANISHI, Y.; KITAHARA, A., and OHTAKE, S.: A possible mechanism of central actions of trazodone in rats. This Symposium (1973).

Author's address: Prof. L. ANGELUCCI, Istituto di Farmacologia e Farmacognosia, University of Rome, *Rome* (Italy)

Toxicology Session
Chairman: A. Hajdu

Trazodone. Mod. Probl. Pharmacopsychiat., vol. 9, pp. 76–86,
ed. Th. A. Ban, Montreal, Que., and B. Silvestrini, Rome (Karger, Basel 1974)

Toxicology of Trazodone

Keith F. Rivett and Patrizio Scorza Barcellona

Huntingdon Research Centre, Huntingdon and Laboratori di Ricerca Farmacologica e Tossicologica ACRAF S.p.A., Rome

Toxicological investigations on trazodone were started some years ago when pharmacological results suggested a potential interest in this drug [Silvestrini *et al.*, 1968]. As the clinical trials corroborated the therapeutic activity of the drug, toxicity studies were extended in duration and enlarged in different laboratories [Scorza Barcellona and Silvestrini, 1967; Scorza Barcellona, 1970; Rivett and Edwards, 1971; Rivett *et al.*, 1971, 1973 a, b; Chesterman and Edwards, 1973; Suzuki, 1973]. However, only a few of these studies have been published. Since trazodone is at the moment under extensive clinical use or experimentation, it appeared useful to review toxicological studies and to present a general picture of the toxicology of this drug.

Results

Acute Toxicity

The acute toxicity of trazodone was studied in mice, rats, rabbits and dogs. Results obtained following intravenous and oral administration are summarized in table I.

The LD_{50} by the i. v. route is 91 mg/kg both in mice and rats, whilst in rabbits the drug is more toxic. In dogs no lethal effect was observed up to 40 mg/kg, which is the maximum amount soluble in a volume of water tolerated by dogs. In subsequent experiments dogs received a total of 60 or 120 mg/kg by injecting 10 or 20 mg/kg every hour. Even with these doses no lethal effect was detected. By the oral route the LD_{50} is similar in

Table 1. Acute toxicity of trazodone (LD_{50} values in mg/kg)

Route of administration	Mouse	Rat	Rabbit	Dog
Intravenous	91	91	52	> 40
Oral	610	690	560	500

the different species used, ranging between about 500 mg/kg in dogs and 690 mg/kg in rats.

Attempts were also made to determine the LD_{50} in both rats and mice following i. m. and s. c. injection. As a general rule, the drug was less toxic than by the oral route. However, solutions containing more than 20–40 mg/ml were found to be very irritant to the tissues, causing necrosis which prevented absorption. The results obtained by these two routes of administration were therefore considered to be meaningless.

For a better understanding of the effects of trazodone in animals of different ages, the LD_{50} was determined in newborn rats (3 days old) and adults using the i. p. route of injection. The LD_{50} was 187 mg/kg to be compared with a value of 178 mg/kg in adult rats. There is thus no difference in the LD_{50} in newborn and adult rats.

In mice, rats and rabbits, lethal doses produced dyspnoea, salivation, prostration and clonic convulsions. In dogs administration of 10–20 mg/kg i. v. induced an immediate state of prostration accompanied by violent tremors and short-lasting convulsions, but recovery was complete within 10–40 min following administration. Administration of 40 mg/kg provoked immediate clonic convulsions lasting some minutes, followed by a state of prostration during which the animals were very agitated. 30 min following treatment the dogs were able to stand but were very aggressive if approached. After 1.5 h the behaviour of the dogs returned to normal. Following oral administration the same clinical features were observed. These, however, started at least 10 min following administration of the drug and lasted for about 5–6 h, after which, depending on the quantity of trazodone ingested, the animal returned to normal or died; the lowest dose consistently producing such disturbances in behaviour was 50 mg/kg. Finally, it must be observed that during the subsequent two weeks all the dogs which survived treatment showed normal behaviour, good appetite and increase of body weight. Autopsy performed at the end of the second week did not show any pathological alterations.

Chronic Toxicity

Table II reports some results obtained in preliminary tests in which trazodone was given repeatedly, once each day for 1–4 months. In rats, a dose of 100 mg/kg p. o. produced some toxic effects which were detectable after 4 months, but not after 1 month of treatment. A dose of 450 mg/kg p. o. caused some deaths.

There was also evidence to show that the drug is more toxic for male rats than female rats. In dogs the first toxic effect consists of disturbances of the CNS, of which clonic convulsions are the most dramatic. These were seen following 50 mg/kg/day and after 100 mg/kg/day one dog died. However, autopsy did not show any anatomo-pathological alterations. It therefore seems that the toxicity is of a functional type, before it becomes organic.

Further studies were then performed to determine dosage levels which could be well tolerated even with prolonged treatment. These studies were performed in rats and dogs treated with the drug by the oral route for 6 months.

Trazodone was given to rats mixed in the diet at a concentration of 0.1 % (15 males and 15 females) and 0.25 % (25 males and 25 females). There were no obvious reactions to treatment; the rats appeared in good physical condition throughout even though the rate of bodyweight gain in male rats receiving the highest dietary level was slightly slower than that in the controls during the first 5 months.

Haematology and blood chemistry were studied at the end of the experiment and showed no marked differences between the values recorded for control animals and those receiving trazodone. When the rats were killed the gross appearance of all the internal organs was normal, although when the principal organs were weighed it was found that the livers from rats that had received 0.25 % in the diet were significantly heavier than those of the control rats. The weights of the livers from rats that had received the lower dietary level were comparable with those of the control rats.

In the experiment carried out on dogs the drug was administered in gelatin capsules. Two male and two female mongrel dogs were given 25 mg/kg each day, one male and one female were given 5 mg/kg each day and another male and female remained undosed for control purposes. Throughout the whole of the dosing period these dogs appeared to be in good physical condition and no abnormal behaviour was observed. Blood samples for hematology and biochemical investigation were obtained, from

Table II. Main results of some preliminary toxicological investigations

Animal species	Duration of treatment, months	Doses, mg/kg/day p. o.	Toxic-effects
Rat	1	100	none
	1	150	reduction of body weight gain in males
	1	450	reduction of body weight gain in males and 2/10 died
	4	100	reduction of body weight gain and slight liver enlargement in males
Dog	1	50	tremors, vomiting, convulsions
	1	100	tremors, convulsions, 1/2 died on day 22

control animals and from those receiving the highest dosage level, before dosing commenced and again after dosing for 3 and 6 months. Samples of blood were only examined from dogs receiving 5 mg/kg/day during the final month. Here also, there were no marked differences between values for control and treated dogs. At the end of the dosing period the dogs were killed and both macroscopic and microscopic examination of the principal tissues revealed no abnormalities.

These studies thus showed that rats tolerated the equivalent of 200–290 mg/kg/day of trazodone when given in the diet and dogs tolerated 25 mg/kg/day with no obvious ill-effect.

It was thereafter decided to perform extensive toxicity studies. It is required by regulatory authorities that the highest dosage level in long-term studies should produce some adverse effects in order to obtain a better assessment of the safety margin. On the basis of the preliminary and pilot studies, it was decided that in rats 300 mg/kg/day would be a suitable high dosage level, whilst the intermediate and low dosage levels were chosen to be 100 and 30 mg/kg/day. Ophthalmoscopic examinations and laboratory investigations were performed at regular intervals throughout the study.

In rats receiving 30 mg/kg/day no behavioural changes were seen at all. In those receiving 100 mg/kg/day some lethargy, lasting up to 3 h, was seen following dosing during the first week only, and salivation was occasionally seen immediately following dosing during the first 30 weeks. Initially, rats receiving the highest dosage level of 300 mg/kg/day salivated excessively within 5 min of dosing, and became inactive, assuming a prone position. Occasional body tremors were also seen. The animals remained prone for approximately 3 h and then slowly returned to normal. The intensity and duration of these reactions slowly diminished as the study progressed, so that by the end of the first 4 weeks the only reaction to treatment observed was salivation immediately following dosing, and even this sign was not seen after week 30.

Treatment with trazodone did not affect the survival rate since the number of animals dying in both the treated and control groups were similar.

All groups of male rats showed significant retardation in the rate of body weight gain, as did females receiving 100 or 300 mg/kg/day. Measurement of food intake, however, showed that only in males receiving the highest dosage level was there a significant reduction in the quantity of food consumed. Examination of samples of blood and urine from rats receiving the highest dosage level at intervals during the study showed that they were comparable with the samples obtained from control rats, and examination of the eyes revealed no abnormalities.

Interim examination of 10 rats of each sex from each group at the end of the first 6 months of dosing revealed no abnormalities. Similarly, after 18 months there were no dose-related microscopic abnormalities, and considering the differences in body weight minor differences existing between the weights of the principal organs from treated and control rats were considered to be of no biological significance.

It may be concluded that the prolonged administration of high doses of trazodone (about one half of the LD_{50}) produced no organic or biochemical changes that may be detected in the common laboratory tests. The same doses produced obvious pharmacological disturbances, like salivation and prostration and the progressive attenuation of these signs during the dosing period suggests that rats develop a resistance to the drug. Liver enlargement observed in the preliminary and pilot experiments suggests an enzymatic induction which is a very common response of rats to drug administration.

In the chronic toxicity study performed on dogs, the animals were treated for 1 year. Trazodone was administered in gelatin capsules at the dose of 40 mg/kg/day (reduced to 30 mg/kg/day after 8 weeks), 20 and 10 mg/kg/day.

Ophthalmoscopic examinations and laboratory investigations were performed at regular intervals.

At the lowest dosage level of 10 mg/kg/day no abnormal signs were seen that could be attributed to treatment with trazodone. At the dosage level of 20 mg/kg/day one dog, during the 15th week of treatment, was found lying on its stomach with all limbs splayed and breathing rapidly. The animal recovered during that day and remained completely normal for the rest of the experiment. No other effect was seen in dogs receiving 20 mg/kg/day until week 51 when a female dog was unexpectedly found dead. Dogs receiving the highest dosage level of 40 mg/kg/day also appeared to be normal for most of the time although 2 males and 1 female died within the first 8 weeks. Because of the death of these 3 dogs so soon after the start of the experiment, the dosage level was reduced to 30 mg/kg/day during week 9.

During the first 3 weeks the only obvious reaction to treatment in dogs receiving 40 mg/kg/day was some incoordination of the limbs on very isolated occasions, and this continued throughout, even when the dosage level was reduced. However, during week 4 one male and one female were observed to have brief convulsions, and both dogs eventually died, the male during week 5 and the female during week 8. Both dogs convulsed just prior to death. In addition, one further dog, a male, died during week 7 after having been in a collapsed state for 2 days.

Following reduction of the high dose level to 30 mg/kg/day the dogs appeared normal at virtually all times. However, 16 weeks after reducing the dosage one female convulsed prior to being dosed one morning. During the next two days it was agitated, hypersensitive when touched, and appeared dazed. It eventually died 1 h following dosing on the third day. At this time it was lying on the kennel floor when it was observed to exhale loudly and die.

The only other abnormal behaviour observed following the reduction of dosage to 30 mg/kg/day was in a female which became hypersensitive to touch and aggressive during the final 6 months.

There was no general adverse effect on food consumption and body weight gain in dogs receiving trazodone did not differ significantly from that of control dogs. Regular ophthalmoscopic examination of the eyes also revealed no abnormalities.

Samples of blood and urine were obtained from all dogs at intervals during the study for full hematological and biochemical analyses. The results of the hematological investigations were normal for all dogs apart from one dog receiving 20 mg/kg/day which showed a transient anemia between weeks 16 and 24. Blood biochemical investigations and urinalysis also revealed no abnormalities apart from slightly elevated SGPT values in one male and one female receiving 30 mg/kg/day during the final 3 months. These values were not markedly increased, the final values being 62 and 86 Sigma Frankel units respectively in the male and female, whilst our normally accepted upper limit is 50 units.

At the end of the first 6 months, 2 males and 2 females from the control group and the groups receiving 10 or 20 mg/kg/day were killed for interim examination. All the surviving dogs were killed after being dosed for 1 year. No abnormalities that were considered to have resulted from dosage with trazodone were seen during either macroscopic examination or when pieces of the principal tissues from all dogs were examined microscopically, and this was also true for all the dogs that died during the study. In addition, the weights of the principal organs from dogs that had received trazodone were comparable with those of the control dogs.

The chronic toxicity study in dogs has been reported in detail since it represents the most crucial aspect of the toxicology of this drug. In accordance with what was observed in rats, there is a clear-cut predominance of pharmacological disturbances such as convulsions and prostration, with no organic and biochemical alterations. Unlike what occurs in rats, dogs do not seem to adapt to the drug and as a consequence they are easily subject to toxic phenomena even after prolonged treatment. The attenuation of symptoms which was observed when the dosage was reduced suggests, furthermore, that toxicity is manifested when the capability of detoxication is exhausted by excessive dosages of the drug.

Teratology

Some of the results of this section will be presented later in detail by Suzuki.

These studies were carried out on rats and rabbits; the drugs were administered by the oral route during the critical period of organogenesis. The results obtained in rats are summarized in table III. A dose of 100 mg/kg/day of trazodone did not bring about embryotoxic effects whereas an evident sedative effect was observed in the mothers. With doses of 150 and 210 mg/kg/day a decrease in the body weight of the mothers was observed as well as an increase in the sedative action. On the other hand, no teratogenic or lethal effect was manifest in the fetuses. A slight delay in the ossification process and a mean fetal weight lower than that of the

Table III. Teratological study in rats

Number and strain of animals	Products, mg/kg/day p. o.	Days of treatment during pregnancy	Toxicity		Terato-genicity, %
			maternal	fetal	
10 Long Evans	trazodone, 100	10–15	±	–	0
18 Wistar	trazodone, 150	9–14	+	+	0
15 Long Evans	trazodone, 210	6–15	+	–	0
18 Wistar	trazodone, 300	9–14	+	+	1
13 Wistar	trazodone, 450	9–14	++	+	1
14 Wistar	imipramine, 150	9–14	++	+	5
14 Long Evans	cyclizine, 75	10–15	+	++	17
9 Long Evans	cyclizine, 100	10–15	+	+++	50

control animals was noted when dosages of 150 mg/kg were administered. The first embryotoxic effects of trazodone were manifested with doses sublethal for the maternal organism; 300 and 450 mg/kg/day bringing about a significant increase of resorptions and the appearance of a minimal percentage of fetal malformations.

At doses of 150 mg/kg/day imipramine used for reference purposes brought about an evident sedative effect in the mothers as well as a cessation of body weight gain; in the fetuses it provoked an increase in the death rate and the appearance of 6 malformed fetuses.

Cyclizine, at doses of 75 and 100 mg/kg/day, exerted a clear-cut embryotoxic action which was shown by a marked increase in resorptions and the appearance of numerous malformed fetuses.

Table IV summarizes the results obtained in rabbits. At a dose of 100 mg/kg/day trazodone exerted an evident sedative action on the mothers, whereas it did not have any embryotoxic effects on the fetuses. At a dosage of 150 mg/kg/day lethargy was observed in the mothers as well as an increase of fetal mortality with respect to the control animals. No teratogenic effects were observed, however. With dosages of 450 mg/kg/day (a sublethal dose for the adult animal) a reduction in the body weight of the fetuses was observed, as compared to the controls; as well as an increase in the death rate; furthermore, one fetus had no tail.

At a dose of 150 mg/kg/day diazepam brought about a deep lethargic

Table IV. Teratological study in rabbits

Number and strain of animals	Products, mg/kg/day p. o.	Days of treatment during pregnancy	Toxicity		Terato-genicity, %
			maternal	fetal	
10 New Zealand white	trazodone, 100	5–18	+	–	0
8 Japanese white	trazodone, 150	8–15	+	+	0
7 Japanese white	trazodone, 450	8–15	+	+	3
8 Japanese white	diazepam, 150	8–15	+	+	0
10 New Zealand white	thalidomide, 100	5–18	–	++	19

state in the mothers as well as a cessation of body weight gain; even the fetuses weighed less than the controls. An increase of fetal mortality was also observed.

Finally, at doses of 100 mg/kg, thalidomide exerted its typical teratogenic activity by provoking serious malformations in 19% of the fetuses without altering significantly the fetal mortality rate as compared to the controls.

In the above studies trazodone exerted no specific teratogenic effect, such as that brought about by cyclizine and thalidomide. Furthermore, it must be remembered that a drug is considered teratogenic if it produces fetal malformations – within a broad dose range – without exerting toxic actions on the maternal organism, and without causing the death of the embryo [SAXÉN and RAPOLA, 1969]. In the case of trazodone the first toxic effects were encountered in the mothers and not in the fetuses. Furthermore, in rabbits, an increase of fetal mortality preceded the appearance of malformations. It must be noted that these latter appeared very rarely and only when very high dosages were administered.

On the basis of the experimental results here reported and the clinical experience gathered so far, there seems to be no particular contraindications for the use of trazodone in women in the reproductive age, except those which are commonly indicated with the use of all drugs.

Conclusions

On the basis of the experiments reported, the picture of trazodone toxicology may be described as follows:

The drug proved to be well tolerated in rats, even in long-term experiments and at doses corresponding to about half the LD_{50}. In fact, these studies did not show any sign of degenerative lesions on organs or tissues or lethal effects. The only sign of toxicity present in rats was prostration which, however, occurred only during the initial period of treatment.

In dogs the acute toxicity of trazodone was the same as that observed in rats, and chronic toxicity tests confirmed the absence of anatomo-pathological lesions and alterations in the hematological tests or blood chemistry.

During these experiments the main toxicological characteristic of trazodone was clearly defined, i. e. the capacity to induce functional disturbances mainly of the CNS. These disturbances can be very severe in dogs and culminate in a convulsive state resulting in death. This effect was observed starting from the fourth week of treatment and only at the higher dosage levels. The toxic effects in dogs receded, or were reduced when the dosage was lowered. Finally the studies conducted on pregnant rats and rabbits, up to sublethal doses, excluded a teratogenic activity of trazodone.

The request of the regulatory authorities, according to whom the highest dosage level in long-term studies should produce some adverse effects, was satisfied indicating the main risk in the therapeutic use of trazodone was, namely, the onset of CNS disturbances such as convulsions and prostration.

Regarding the margin between the therapeutic doses in human and the toxic doses in animals the following observations can be made. The rat tolerated well the prolonged administration of 300 mg/kg/day of trazodone. On the contrary, dogs proved to tolerate well only lower dosages, namely 10 mg/kg/day for 1 year and of 25 mg/kg/day for 6 months; therefore the use of the drug in humans will be discussed in connection with toxicity in the dog, which is more sensitive to trazodone.

The common human dosage level, mostly used in psychoneuroses, is 25 mg three times daily, i. e. approximately 1.3 mg/kg/day. There should, therefore, be no problem associated with this dosage regime in man since the no-effect dosage level in the dog is at least 8 times as great. However, in more severe diseases, like depressive states, trazodone was found effective in higher doses, ranging between 50 and 200 mg three times daily, i. e.

up to 10 mg/kg/day. From the results in the dog study it would appear that a consistent risk is attached to this regime. Nevertheless, it should be pointed out that clinical experience in this regard allows us to affirm that trazodone has not produced any toxic effects worthy of note or at any rate comparable to those observed in the dog.

References

CHESTERMAN, H. and EDWARDS, D. B.: Trazodone acute toxicity in beagle dogs. Intravenous and oral dosage. Personal commun. (1973).

RIVETT, K. F.; BATHAM, P., and SPICER, E. J. F.: Preliminary trazodone toxicity study in rats. Oral administration for 4 weeks. Personal commun. (1971).

RIVETT, K. F.; CHESTERMAN, H.; EDWARDS, D. B.; STREET, A. E., and NEWMAN, A. J.: Trazodone – oral toxicity study in beagle dogs. Repeated dosage for one year. Personal commun. (1973 a).

RIVETT, K. F. and EDWARDS, D. B.: Trazodone – initial toxicity study in beagle dogs. Personal commun. (1971).

RIVETT, K. F.; HUNTER, B.; BATHAM, P.; STREET, A. E.; HEYWOOD, R., and CHERRY, C. P.: Trazodone – oral toxicity to rats. Repeated administration for 78 weeks with interim sacrifice at 26 weeks. Personal commun. (1973 b).

SAXEN, L. and RAPOLA, J.: Congenital deffects. Developmental biology, p. 184 (Holt, Rinehart & Winston, New York 1969).

SCORZA BARCELLONA, P.: Investigations on the possible teratogenic effects of Trazodone in rats and rabbits. Boll. chim. farm. *109:* 323–332 (1970).

SCORZA BARCELLONA, P. e SILVESTRINI, B.: Ricerche tossicologiche sull'AF 1161, un nuovo farmaco psicotropo. Personal commun. (1967).

SILVESTRINI, B.; CIOLI, V.; BURBERI, S., and CATANESE, B.: Pharmacological properties of AF 1161, a new psychotropic drug. Int. J. Neuropharmacol. *7:* 587–599 (1968).

SUZUKI, Y.: Teratogenicity and placental transfer of trazodone. This volume (1973).

Author's address: K. F. RIVETT, Huntingdon Research Centre, *Huntingdon* (England)

Trazodone. Mod. Probl. Pharmacopsychiat., vol. 9, pp. 87–94,
ed. Th. A. Ban, Montreal, Que., and B. Silvestrini, Rome (Karger, Basel 1974)

Teratogenicity and Placental Transfer of Trazodone

YOSHIKAZU SUZUKI

Toxicological and Experimental Biology Research Laboratories, Division of Research and Development, Eisai Co. Ltd., Tokyo

Introduction

A teratological study of trazodone in rats and rabbits has been reported by SCORZA BARCELLONA [1970]. This study was also conducted to determine the teratogenic potential of trazodone in rats and rabbits, but different strains and higher dosages were used. In addition, we studied maternal-embryonic transfer of trazodone in rats (after a single administration) in early pregnancy.

Teratogenicity in Rats

Teratogenicity of trazodone in mature Wistar rats was compared with that of imipramine.

The dose levels of 150, 300 or 450 mg/kg/day of trazodone and 150 mg/kg/day of imipramine as a reference drug were used. Drugs were administered by gavage from day 9 to 14 of gestation. Body weights were measured during gestation. The number of implantations, live and dead fetuses were recorded. Fetuses were weighed and examined for external, visceral and skeletal anomalies (table I).

The degree of lethargy, hypomotility and salivation were related to the dose levels of trazodone and imipramine after every administration. Hyposthenia and death were found in the 450 mg/kg trazodone and in the imipramine groups. Body weight gain of dams at the dose levels of 150 and 300 mg/kg were slightly decreased, but in the 450 mg/kg trazodone and in the imipramine groups they were significantly decreased.

Table I. Effects of trazodone on rat fetuses after oral administration on days 9–14 of gestation

	Control	Trazodone, mg/kg			Imi-pramine, 150 mg/kg
		150	300	450	
Mothers					
Number of examined	20	18	18	16	17
Number of dead	0	0	0	3[1]	3[2]
Body weight gains, g	114	100	97	73[1]	36[1]
Fetuses					
At term					
Mean implant.	13.9	13.9	14.5	13.7	13.4
Resorb. and dead, %	5.0	7.6	15.0[1]	25.3[1]	34.0[1]
Mean live fetuses	13.2	12.9	12.3[1]	10.2[1]	8.8[1]
Mean weight, g	3.60	3.39[1]	3.16[1]	2.91[1]	2.87[1]
Ossification					
Undeveloped					
Sternebrae, %	5.1	7.6	11.5[2]	25.8[1]	22.2[1]
Metacarpals, %	26.6	68.8[1]	96.6[1]	80.9[1]	84.0[1]
Unossified prox. of forelimb, %	37.3	73.2[1]	94.6[1]	78.7[1]	93.8[1]
Mean number of caudal	3.4	3.2	2.7[1]	2.2[1]	2.7[2]

1, 2 Significant at 1- and 5-percent levels, respectively, as compared with control.

These findings are in accord with those observed in acute and subacute toxicity studies [TANAKA, 1973; SUGIYAMA, 1973; RIVETT *et al.*, 1973]. Therefore, these changes in the dams seem to be ascribed to large doses of drugs. The effects encountered in the 450 mg/kg trazodone group were of a lower degree than those observed in the dams of the imipramine group.

The fetal mortality increase was dose-related with both trazodone and imipramine. Fetal weights in the trazodone-treated groups showed a dose-related decrease, while in the imipramine group these effects were lower if compared with the 450 mg/kg of trazodone group. Retardation of ossifications were observed along with fetal weight decrease.

The occurrence of fetal mortality and retardation of fetal development, such as less gain of body weight, hyposthenia and suppression of food consumption could be attributed to maternal toxicity; these findings were also

Table II. Number and types of malformations observed among rat fetuses after oral administration of trazodone on day 9–14 of gestation

	Control	Trazodone, mg/kg			Imi-pramine, 150 mg/kg
		150	300	450	
External					
Number of examined	265	232	222	133	124
Umbilical hernia	0	0	3	1	0
Exencephalia	0	0	0	1	0
Ectrodactylia	0	0	0	0	2
Deviation of digits	0	0	0	0	2
Syndactyly	0	0	0	0	2
Number of examined for internal.	88	75	74	44	43
Anomalies	0	0	0	0	0
Skeletal					
Number of examined	177	157	148	89	81
Lumbar rib	7	14	2	1	1
Abnormal sternebrae	2	1	0	0	0
Branched rib	0	0	1	0	0
Waved rib	0	0	0	0	1
Separated thoracic arch	0	0	1	2	0

observed in the subacute toxicity studies (table II) [SUGIYAMA, 1973; RIVETT *et al.*, 1973].

In external anomalies, umbilical hernia, exencephalia, ectrodactylia, deviation of digits and syndactylia were found in one or three fetuses. In regard to skeletal findings lumbar rib and abnormal vertebrae were found in all groups while other anomalies, such as branched or waved rib and separated thoracic body, were found in one or two fetuses. No anomalies were found in the visceral organs.

It has been known that umbilical hernia and separated thoracic arch of fetus is associated with retardation of fetal development. Besides, the incidence of such anomalies was low and found in only 1 or 2 fetuses of 1 or 2 dams in all groups.

Thus, it is concluded that trazodone and imipramine had no direct teratogenic effects on the rat fetuses, since adverse effects were only noted at such large doses as required for inducing maternal toxicity.

Table III. Effects of trazodone on rabbit fetuses after oral administration on day 8–15 of gestation

	Control	Trazodone, mg/kg		Diazepam, 150 mg/kg
		150	450	
Mothers				
Number of examined	8	8	7	8
Body weight gains, g	670	520[2]	540[2]	470[1]
At term				
Mean implant.	8.6	7.6	7.4	9.4
Resorb. and dead, %	5.8	14.8[2]	34.6[1]	14.7[2]
Mean live fetuses	8.1	6.5[2]	4.9[1]	8.0[2]
Mean weight, g	37.1	37.9	31.5[2]	31.8[2]
Crown-rump length, cm	7.56	7.56	7.03[2]	7.28
Tail length, cm	1.40	1.46	1.25	1.35
Fetuses				
Ossification				
Reduced skull ossification, %	52.3	57.8	90.6[1]	34.6
Undeveloped mid. digits of				
Forelimb, %	13.8	37.5[1]	37.5[1]	9.6
Hindlimb, %	1.5	17.2[1]	9.4[2]	3.8

1, 2 Significant at 5% levels as compared with control.

Teratogenicity in Rabbits

Teratogenic effects of trazodone in mature Japanese white rabbits were studied in comparison with diazepam.

Dose levels of 150 or 450 mg/kg/day of trazodone and 150 mg/kg/day of diazepam as a reference drug were used. Drugs were administered by gavage from day 8 to 15 of gestation. The fetuses were delivered by cesarean section on day 29 of gestation. The number of implantations and live or dead fetuses were determined. Fetuses were weighed and examined for viability, external and internal skeletal anomalies (table III).

Lethargy and hypomotility were related to the dose levels in treated dams after every administration. The body weight gains of dams were decreased in each treated group.

Table IV. Effects of trazodone and diazepam on survivals of incubated fetuses from rabbits after oral administration on day 8–15 of gestation

	Control	Trazodone, mg/kg		Diazepam, 150 mg/kg
		150	450	
Number of fetuses				
Alive at term	65	52	34	64
Survivals after 24 h	49	27	14	29
Dead within 24 h, %	24.6	48.1[1]	58.8[1]	54.6[1]
Time dead				
> 1 h	4	0	10	24[1]
> 6 h	11	10	1	7
> 24 h	1	15[1]	9[1]	4

1 Significant at the 1-percent level as compared with control.

These results were in accord with the above-mentioned results from teratological studies and other subacute toxicity studies in rats [SUGIYAMA, 1973; RIVETT *et al.*, 1973]. These findings in dams were more marked in the diazepam group than in the 450 mg/kg trazodone group.

Incidence of the fetal mortality was recorded in the trazodone and diazepam-treated groups. Fetal weight was decreased in the 450 mg/kg and diazepam groups; crown-rump and tail length also tended to be shorter in those groups. Ossifications were retarded only in the trazodone-treated groups (table IV).

The survival time of the incubated fetuses was shorter in the treated groups than in the control group. These developmental retardations of fetuses such as lethargy, hypomotility and body weight decrease seem to be a consequence of maternal toxicity (table V).

There were no internal or external anomalies except one absent tail in the 450 mg/kg group. In the skeletal anomalies lumbar ribs were found in all groups including the control group. But the incidence of this anomaly was not related to the dose levels.

Therefore, it was concluded from this study that trazodone was not teratogenic in the rabbits. It seems that fetal mortality, developmental retardation of live fetuses and lesser viability of incubated fetuses in the treated groups were attributed to maternal toxicity.

Table V. Number and types of malformation observed among rabbit fetuses after oral administration of trazodone on day 8–15 of gestation

	Control	Trazodone, mg/kg		Diazepam, 150 mg/kg
		150	450	
Number of examined	65	52	34	64
Absent tail	0	0	1	0
Internal anomalies	0	0	0	0
Lumbar rib	37	24[2]	20	11[1]

1, 2 Significant at the 5- and 1-percent levels, respectively, as compared with control.

Maternal-Embryonic Transfer in Rats

The maternal-embryonic transfer in rats was studied. Trazodone was given orally to Wistar rats on day 14 of gestation at the dose of 150 mg/kg. Maternal blood, litter of embryos and amnion were collected at various time intervals after drug administration. In these samples, we measured the amount of trazodone by CATANESE's spectrophotofluorimetric method (fig. 1) [CATANESE and LISCIANI, 1970].

Levels of trazodone in maternal blood was increased up to 10 min, then decreased gradually and reached the lowest level 720 min after drug administration.

The drug levels in a litter of embryos were always lower than those in maternal blood. The peak levels in embryos appeared 5 min later than that in maternal blood. The amnion levels were lower than those in maternal blood and embryos. In fact even the highest level of drug in amnion (detected 15–30 min following administration) could barely be measured.

From the results mentioned above, it would appear that trazodone, given to the pregnant rats, was minimally transferred to embryos.

Conclusion

The investigations of teratogenic potential and placental transfer of trazodone in laboratory animals, showed no teratogenic effects on rat and

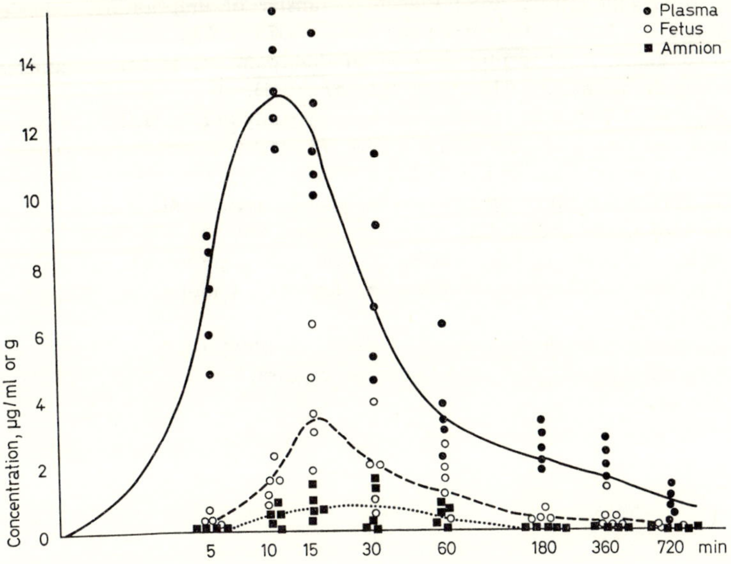

Fig. 1. Placental transfer of trazodone in rats after a single oral administration.

rabbit fetuses. Although fetal mortality and growth retardation in live fetuses were noticed, these embryotoxic effects were more marked in the imipramine and diazepam groups than in the trazodone-treated groups. Similar teratological findings of trazodone in rats and rabbits have been reported by SCORZA BARCELLONA [1970].

In maternal-embryonic transfer studies of trazodone in rats, it was found that the drug was minimally transferred to embryos. Placental transfer of imipramine in rats and diazepam in mice have been reported by DOUGLAS and HOME [1967] and IDÄNPÄÄN-HEIKKILA [1971].

Effects observed in embryos could be attributed to either placental transfer of trazodone or maternal toxicity or both. It is concluded that trazodone has less toxic effects in embryos than imipramine or diazepam.

References

CATANESE, B. and LISCIANI, R.: Investigation on the absorption and distribution of trazodone or AF 1161 in rats, dogs and humans. Boll. chim. farm. *109:* 369–373 (1970).

DOUGLAS, B. H. and HUME, A. S.: Placental transfer of imipramine, a basic, lipid soluble drug. Amer. J. Obstet. Gynec. *99:* 573–575 (1967).

IDÄNPÄÄN-HEIKKILA, J.: Placental transfer of diazepam ^{14}C in mice, hamsters and monkeys J. Pharm. exp. Ther. *176:* 752–757 (1971).

RIVETT, K., *et al.:* I. Preliminary trazodone toxicity study in rats. II. Trazodone toxicity to rats repeated oral administration for 78 weeks. Intern. report (Huntingdon Research Center, Huntingdon, London 1973).

SCORZA BARCELLONA, P.: Investigations on the possible teratogenic effects of trazodone or AF 1161 in rats and rabbits. Boll. chim. farm. *109:* 323–332 (1970).

SUGIYAMA, K.: Subacute toxicity studies of oral trazodone in rats. Internal Report (Toxicology and Experimental Biology Research Laboratories, Eisai Co. Ltd., Tokyo 1973).

TANAKA, S.: Acute toxicological tests of trazodone. Internal Report (Toxicology and Experimental Biology Research Laboratories, Eisai Co. Ltd., Tokyo 1973).

Author's address: YOSHIKAZU SUZUKI, Toxicological and Experimental Biology Research Laboratories, Divison of Research and Development, Eisai Co. Ltd., Koishikawa 4, Bunkyo, *Tokyo* (Japan)

First Clinical Session

Chairman: C. CAZZULO

Trazodone. Mod. Probl. Pharmacopsychiat., vol. 9, pp. 95–109,
ed. Th. A. Ban, Montreal, Que., and B. Silvestrini, Rome (Karger, Basel 1974)

Trazodone – A Review of Literature

J. SAARMA

Laboratory of Psychopharmacology, Department of Psychiatry, State University, Tartu

Remarks on the History of Trazodone

Trazodone, chemically 2-[3-(4-m-chlorophenyl)-1-piperazinyl] propyl s. triazolo[4,3-a]pyridin-3-(2H)one), was synthesized in 1966 by PALAZZO [37] in the chemical laboratories of F. Angelini. Pharmacological studies carried out by SILVESTRINI [45] in 1967 revealed that trazodone has definite CNS activity.

Early clinical studies by BRAVACCIO *et al.* [9] in 1967, by POZZI *et al.* [40] in 1967 and by CIANCHETTI and GAINOTTI [16] in 1968 demonstrated that trazodone has therapeutic action in patients suffering from depressive states, neuroses and some other conditions.

On the basis of these results, trazodone, the first s-triazolo[4,3-a] pyridine derivative ever used in therapy, was introduced into contemporary psychopharmacology [5, 9, 16, 37, 40, 45].

In recent years a great number of clinical investigations on trazodone have been carried out in many countries, particularly in Italy and in Canada. These studies have confirmed that trazodone possesses certain antidepressant and antianxiety action and has some advantages in comparison with already known psychotropic drugs.

At the 2nd Meeting of the International College of Psychosomatic Medicine, held in Amsterdam in June 1973, a Round Table Discussion on trazodone presented new data on the therapeutic application of the drug [49, 50].

The present First International Symposium on Trazodone, in Montreal, may be regarded as an expression of the great interest which psychiatrists, pharmacologists and other specialists have in this drug.

Table I. Some pharmacological properties of trazodone in comparison with sedatives and neuroleptics according to SILVESTRINI [45], SILVESTRINI and LISCIANI [46] and SILVESTRINI and QUADRI [47]

Variables	Sedatives	Neuroleptics	Trazodone
Spontaneous motor activity	–	–	–
Hexobarbital-induced sleep	+	+	+
Analgesic activity	+	+	+
Two neuronal reflex	0	–	0
Multi-neuronal reflex	–	0	–
Body temperature	0	–	0
Cataleptogenic effect	0	+	0
Anti-apomorphine effect	0	+	0
Anti-convulsant effect	+	0	0
Conditional avoidance reflex	0	–	–
Amphetamine group toxicity	0	–	(–)
Anti-noradrenaline effect	0	+	+
Anti-serotonine effect	0	+	+
Anti-histamine effect	0	+	±
Anti-acetylcholine effect	0	+	±
Anti-L-dopa effect	0	+	±

The task of the following presentation is to review the studies on trazodone which have been published to date.

Pharmacological Studies

A. Animal Pharmacology

A considerable number of pharmacological studies on trazodone have been carried out in animals [12–14, 21, 23, 45–47].

SILVESTRINI [45] already pointed out in his first publication on trazodone in 1967 that pharmacological properties of this compound are quite different from the actions of known types of psychotropic drugs. Some features of trazodone are similar to tranquilizers, while other effects are different (table I). At the same time, some actions of trazodone are common with neuroleptics, but some other features are quite different. SILVESTRINI

Table II. Some pharmacological properties of trazodone in comparison with antidepressants (according to SILVESTRINI and LISCIANI [46])

	Anti-depressants	Trazodone
Anti-MAO effect	+	0
Anti-reserpine effect	+	0
Catecholamine-potentiating effect	+	0
5HT-potentiating effect	+	0
Activation of amygdala's after-discharge	+	±

pointed out that trazodone obviously possesses the property to selectively act on the mechanisms of integration and emotional elaboration of painful stimuli and, generally speaking, of the stimuli capable of activating emotogenic systems [45, 46]. Therefore, he concluded trazodone may be recommended in depressive and anxiety conditions. It is well known that further clinical experience has confirmed SILVESTRINI'S prediction.

Paradoxically, pharmacological studies, at the same time, have demonstrated that trazodone does not bring about most of the effects regarded as typical for antidepressants (table II).

It must be pointed out that the mechanism of action as well as exact pharmacological characteristics of trazodone are still awaiting to be established. On the other hand, it has been impossible to classify trazodone on the basis of its pharmacological properties in accordance with the generally recognized classification of psychotropic drugs.

B. Human Pharmacology

The pharmacological effects of trazodone in man have been dealt with in a limited number of studies.

CATANESE and LISCIANI [14] established that the highest blood concentration of trazodone in man is reached two hours after oral administration. There is no more trazodone in the blood after 24 h.

Apart from the small amount excreted through the kidneys, most of the trazodone undergoes metabolic changes, the nature of which is not precisely known.

CONTI *et al.* [18] and MAGGINI *et al.* [34] carried out investigations by means of sleep EEG recording. They found that trazodone brings about an increase in the total sleep time and a decrease in re-awakenings, with some decrease of stage I and increase of stage II of sleep. They could not find any changes, typical either of other thymoleptics (decrease of REM, increase of stage IV) or of tranquilizers (increase of REM, decrease of stage IV). These findings once again stress the unique properties of trazodone, as compared with other psychotropic drugs.

BAN and LEHMANN [6] and BAN *et al.* [7] have studied the action of trazodone in normal persons by means of psychophysical tests (Verdun Psychometric Test Battery). They found that auditory reaction time, tapping speed, track tracer time and cancellation test errors improved, while critical flicker fusion frequency decreased under the effect of trazodone. From these results, BAN and co-workers draw the conclusion that trazodone brings about an increase in perceptual input and an improvement in integrative processing as well as in psychomotor performance, thereby facilitating the restoration of the balance between arousal and integration. On the basis of these considerations, it has been suggested that trazodone may be effective in patients suffering from organic brain syndrome [6, 7, 35].

Clinical Studies

A considerable number of clinical studies carried out with trazodone have suggested various possibilities for the therapeutic applications of this compound.

A. Efficacy of Trazodone

1. Trazodone in Depressive States

Starting from the first clinical investigations by BRAVACCIO *et al.* [9], POZZI *et al.* [40], CIANCHETTI and GAINOTTI [16] the marked antidepressive action of trazodone has been demonstrated (table III), both in uncontrolled and double-blind placebo-controlled studies. In standard controlled studies the antidepressive efficacy – 50 to 80 % in different samples – has been found to be equal to amitriptyline [16, 51] and imipramine [17, 31].

There is, however, a diversity of opinions concerning the type of depression most favourably responding to trazodone. In some studies trazo-

Table III. Trazodone in depressive states

Author(s)	Year	Number of patients on trazodone	Percentage of remissions	General conclusion
BRAVACCIO *et al.* [9]	1967	17	n. a.	effective especially in endogenous depression without anxiety
POZZI *et al.* [40]	1967	17	50	effective especially in endogenous depression without anxiety
CIANCHETTI and GAINOTTI [16]	1968	37	50	equal to amitriptyline
DE GREGORIO and DIONISIO [30]	1969	285	50	effective in all depressions especially without anxiety
DI GIUSEPPE and CESARINI [27]	1969	11	80	effective especially in patients without anxiety
CONTI *et al.* [18]	1969	20	75	effective especially in patients with anxiety
TANSELLA and DELLA RUSSO [48]	1969	14	50	effective especially in patients with sluggishness
CIOFFI *et al.* [17]	1969	12	40	equal to imipramine
MAGGINI *et al.* [34]	1969	6	n. a.	effective in patients with anxiety
DI GIUSEPPE and DIONISIO [28]	1970	9	65	effective also in patients with anxiety
DE GREGORIO and DIONISIO [31]	1971	37	60	equal to imipramine
PARIANTE [38]	1971	17	70	effective especially in patients with apathy
VINCI [51]	1971	33	75	equal to amitriptyline
BAN *et al.* [7]	1973	10	80	effective in depression [2]
AMIN *et al.* [2]	1973	10	80	effective in depression [7]
Total		525	40–80	antidepressive action established

done was found to be most effective in endogenous depressions [9, 40]. In other samples best results were achieved in psychogenic depressions [18, 28, 30]. Some authors have pointed out that trazodone is particularly effective in depression without anxiety [9, 27, 30, 40] or even in retarded and/or apathetic depressions [38, 48]. On the other hand, in some studies best results have been obtained in patients with anxious depression [18, 34].

There are also some studies where the therapeutic effect of trazodone was found to be equal in depressions both with and without anxiety [2, 7, 28]. AMIN *et al.* [2] and BAN *et al.* [7], using multiple rating scales, have pointed out that trazodone brings about an improvement in both anxiety and apathy scores.

In all studies a rapid onset – usually within 3 to 7 days – of the therapeutic action of trazodone has been stressed.

The average dosage applied in depressive states is 300–500 mg p.o. daily, divided into three or four doses. Some investigators prefer to start with smaller dosages (100–150 mg daily) with gradual increments up to 500–600 mg daily. AMIN *et al.* [2] and BAN *et al.* [7] have found that a daily dosage of 75 mg is sufficient to obtain optimal therapeutic effects. Their finding was that further dosage did not enhance results, although this point needs to be further substantiated.

2. Trazodone in Anxiety States

The anti-anxiety action of trazodone has been investigated in different psychogenic as well as somatogenic conditions.

a) Neurotic anxiety states. BRAVACCIO *et al.* [9] as well as TANSELLA and DELLO RUSSO [48] could not establish an anti-anxiety action of trazodone (table IV). In other clinical trials, however, a good tranquilizing effect of trazodone was encountered, equal or even superior to standard tranquilizers [4, 29, 39]. GENTILI and DIONISIO [25] even concluded that the anti-anxiety action of trazodone is superior to the antidepressive effect.

In this connection it must be pointed out that in most of the studies where favourable anti-anxiety results have been noticed, trazodone was administered in daily dosages of 75 mg. In studies with unfavourable results the dosages applied were much higher [9, 48]. It would be worthwhile to carry out special studies designed to establish optimal dosage.

The finding reported by BARTILOTTI and DIONISIO [8] is highly interesting for further clinical trials – that in acute spells of anxiety a single intravenous administration of trazodone (50 mg) may bring about an excellent therapeutic effect.

b) Somatogenic anxiety states. Trazodone has been administered in a number of patients suffering from various somatic diseases (cardiac, pulmonary, gastrointestinal, etc.) complicated by anxiety states (table V). In

Table IV. Trazodone in neurotic anxiety states

Author(s)	Year	Number of patients on trazodone	Percentage of remissions	General conclusion
Bravaccio *et al.* [9]	1967	7	n. a.	not effective
Tansella and Dello Russo [48]	1969	8	n. a.	not effective
Gentili and Dionisio [25]	1969	37	60	anti-anxiety effect superior to anti-depressive effect
Maggini *et al.* [34]	1969	6	n. a.	good anti-anxiety effect
De Gregorio [29]	1971	179	45	equal to diazepam
Pennesi [39]	1971	19	60	superior to chlordiazepoxide
Argenta [4]	1972	29	70	superior to chlordiazepoxide
Bartilotti and Dionisio [8]		48	95	excellent anti-anxiety effect (especially intravenously)
Antonelli *et al.* [3]	1973	15	75	good anti-anxiety effect
Total		348	45–95	anti-anxiety action established

Table V. Trazodone in somatogenic anxiety states

Author(s)	Year	Number of patients on trazodone	Percentage of remissions	General conclusion
Bufalari [10]	1972	25	95	excellent anti-anxiety effect
Corea [19]		25	90	excellent anti-anxiety effect
Pretolani [41]	1972	40	90	excellent anti-anxiety and hypnotic effect
Gunella and Melica [32]	1973	28	n. a.	good anti-anxiety effect, does not supress respiratory center
Knobel [33]	1973	68	80	good anti-anxiety effect
Total		186	80–95	anti-anxiety effect in psychosomatic conditions established

Table VI. Trazodone as premedication in surgical and other procedures

Author(s)	Year	Condition when trazodone applied	Number of patients	General conclusion
DIONISIO *et al.* [22]	1971	gynecological procedures	50	good sedative effect
SIGNORE *et al.* [44]	1971	gynecological procedures	50	excellent sedative and partly analgesic effect
ALTISSIMI *et al.* [1]	1971	preanesthesia in cesarean section	70	excellent sedative effect
REGGIANI *et al.* [42]	1972	urological endoscopy	43	excellent sedative and partly analgesic effect
BUOMPADRE *et al.* [11]	1972	preanesthesia in surgery	20	good sedative effect
RUGGIERO *et al.* [43]	1973	preanesthesia in surgery	20	superior to haloperidol
GERARDI [26]	1973	preanesthesia in surgery	28	synergistic with relaxants
VINCI and IACOMETTA [52]	1973	premedication in ECT	14	synergistic with succinylcholine and ECT
Total			295	effective as sedative premedication

all studies a good tranquilizing effect has been noted. It must be pointed out that trazodone in dosages of 50–75 mg p. o. is very well tolerated by somatic patients and no marked adverse reactions in these samples have been encountered. GUNELLA and MELICA [32] used trazodone in patients with severe respiratory insufficiency and pointed out that no signs of suppression of respiratory functions were found.

c) Preoperational anxiety states. Beginning in 1971 trazodone has been applied in dosages of 50 mg i. m. or i. v. as premedication in surgical and other (gynecological, endoscopy, etc.) procedures (table VI). All investigators unanimously report a marked sedative effect [1, 11, 22, 43], which seems to be combined with a certain analgesic effect [42, 44] and/or

Table VII. Trazodone in schizophrenia

Author(s)	Year	Number of patients on trazodone	Percentage of remissions	General conclusion
BRAVACCIO *et al.* [9]	1967	10	n. a.	not effective
DE GREGORIO and DIONISIO [30]	1969	100	25	no antipsychotic effect
TANSELLA and DELLO RUSSO [48]	1969	14	50	no antipsychotic effect; effective in defect
DI GIUSEPPE and DIONISIO [28]	1970	6	65	slightly inferior to chlorpromazine
BAN *et al.* [7]	1973	10	50	no antipsychotic effect [24]
GALVAN *et al.* [24]	1973	10	50	no antipsychotic effect [7]
Total		140	25–65	antipsychotic action not established

with synergic effect with muscle relaxants [26, 52]. Lack of interaction with anticoagulants [20] can be regarded as a favourable feature of trazodone when applied in preanesthesia.

An interesting finding is reported by VINCI and IACOMETTA [52] who administered trazodone as premedication before ECT procedures. They found that trazodone produced not only a good tranquilizing effect, but also potentiated the action of succinylcholine and obviously contributed to enhancing the overall efficacy of ECT.

3. Trazodone in Schizophrenia

Up to present time clinical experience with trazodone in schizophrenic patients – scarce as it is – has not been favourable (table VII). Only DI GIUSEPPE and DIONISIO [28] concluded that the efficacy of trazodone is only slightly inferior to chlorpromazine. All other investigators have found that trazodone does not have any antipsychotic effect in schizophrenic patients. Nevertheless, taking into consideration that some minor anti-L-dopa activity of trazodone has been revealed [46] it would be worth carrying out further studies in this direction, applying higher dosages of trazodone. Also, some favourable effects in defective withdrawn schizophrenics, reported by TANSELLA and DELLO RUSSO [48], may stimulate further trials in these patient classifications.

4. Trazodone in Geriatric Patients

There are only three studies dealing with the effect of trazodone in geriatric patients (table VIII). CEINO [15] and PACIARONI [36] noted good sedative and some mood-elevating effects in geriatic patients, but no therapeutic shifts in disorientation and memory disturbance were observed.

BAN *et al.* [7] and NAIR *et al.* [35] have put forward an original hypothesis. They postulate that trazodone may have a positive influence on the integrative (processing) functions and thereby facilitate the restoration of the balance between arousal and integration.

B. Tolerance and Side Effects

In all studies an excellent tolerance of trazodone is unanimously reported. Even when applied in high dosages (up to 1,200 mg daily by GENTILI and DIONISIO) and/or for a long time (up to three months by CEINO), trazodone does not bring about any significant unfavourable effect. It has been found to be very well tolerated in geriatric patients, in patients suffering from different serious somatic diseases, from glaucoma and from respiratory insufficiency.

In a great number of studies a total absence of any side-effect has been noted. In more scrupulous investigations [7, 30] a number of different side-effects has been recorded (table IX). As a rule, these side-effects have been encountered in a small number of patients treated with trazodone, mainly only in the beginning of the treatment. In none of these studies were extrapyramidal signs encountered.

All authors agree that side-effects with trazodone are rare, mild and transient, and do not call for discontinuation of treatment.

Clinical Conclusions

Clinical investigations carried out since 1967 have provided enough evidence to conclude that trazodone is endowed with definite psychoactive properties.

A marked antidepressive action of trazodone has been established,

Table VIII. Trazodone in geriatric patients

	Year	Number of patients on trazodone	Percentage of remissions	General conclusion
CEINO [15]	1972	48	55	good effect
PACIARONI [36]	1971	15	70	good effect
BAN *et al.* [7]	1973	10	60	improves mood and organicity [35]
NAIR *et al.* [35]	1973	10	60	improves mood and organicity [7]
Total		73	55–70	

although, it is still not clearly defined in what type of depression the most favourable effects can be expected.

A considerable tranquilizing action has been established. Trazodone has been found to be effective in psychogenic and somatogenic anxiety states, as well as in preanesthesia and in the preparation of patients for 'uncomfortable' diagnostic or therapeutic procedures.

No marked antipsychotic effect of trazodone has been established to date.

Tolerance of trazodone is extremely good. Slight and transient side-effects have been encountered in only a small ratio of patients.

Suggestions for Further Clinical Investigations

It is necessary to carry out controlled studies, using clinico-physiological and psychophysical assessments, in large samples of patients in various psychiatric conditions (similar to designs by BAN and LEHMANN) [6]. Priority aims of these studies should be: (1) to find out differential indications for trazodone, and (2) to find out appropriate dosages of the drug in different conditions.

Special studies could be carried out with trazodone: (1) in withdrawn and apathetic schizophrenics; (2) in depressive patients using intravenous route of administration; (3) in patients with organic brain syndromes (both

Table IX. Side effects under trazodone administration

Behavioral	
	Drowsiness [7, 25, 30, 41]
	Hypersomnia [4, 30]
	Somnolence [30]
	Confusional state [7]
	Increased impulsiveness [30, 48]
	Insomnia [7, 16, 38]
	Anxiety [30, 48]
	Psychomotor agitation [7, 30]
Neurological	
	Dizziness [15, 16, 18, 19, 22, 30, 38]
	Headache [7, 19, 28, 30, 51]
	Tremor [7, 30]
Autonomic	
	Hypotension [1, 9, 28, 30, 38, 40, 43, 48]
	Hypertension [1, 7]
	Tachycardia [7]
	Dryness in mouth [7, 15, 22, 30, 51]
	Nausea [7, 28, 30]
	Constipation [7, 18]
	Diarrhea [7, 51]
Laboratory	
	Anemia (transient) [7]

geriatric and other); and (4) in addicts, especially in alcoholics as maintenance treatment to prevent relapses.

The tolerance and the effect of various combinations of trazodone with other drugs and/or procedures should also be investigated, e. g. combination with ECT in depressive states, with antipsychotic neuroleptics in schizophrenia, with glutamic and/or γ-amino-butyric acid in organic brain syndromes.

References

1 Altissimi, C.; Mastrostefano, M. P. e Signore, L.: Premedicazione anestetica all'intervento per taglio cesareo con AF 1161. Acta anaesth. *22:* 587–598 (1971).

2 AMIN, M.; BAN, T. A., and KLINGNER, A.: Trazodone in the treatment of affective disorders. Current Therapeutic Research *15:* 781–788 (1973).

3 ANTONELLI, F.; DE GREGORIO, M., and DIONISIO, A.: Trazodone in the treatment of psychoneuroses; a double-blind study. Current Therapeutic Research *15:* 799–809 (1973).

4 ARGENTA, G.: Il trittico (trazodone) nella terapia dell'ansia. Policlinico, Sez. med. *79:* 174–180 (1972).

5 BAIOCCHI, L.; CHIARI, A.; FRIGERIO, A., and RIDOFI, P.: Analytical profile of trazodone. Arzneimittelforsch. *23:* 400–406 (1973).

6 BAN, T. A. and LEHMANN, H. E.: Systematic clinical studies with trazodone: methodological aspects. Current Therapeutic Research *15:* 764–769 (1973).

7 BAN, T. A.; LEHMANN, H. E.; AMIN, M.; GALVAN, L.; NAIR, N. P. V.; VERGARA, L., and ZOCH, C.: Comprehensive clinical studies with trazodone. Curr. therap. Res. *15:* 540–551 (1973).

8 BARTILOTTI, R. and DIONISIO, A.: A new minor tranquilizer for the treatment of psychoneurosis (in press).

9 BRAVACCIO, F.; POZZI, O.; MARGHERITA, G. e MASTROSIMONE, F.: Prima esplorazione clinica ed elettroencefalografica degli effetti dell'Af 1161 in pazienti psichiatrici. Comunicazione presentata alla 1ª Riunione naz. della soc. ital. di Neuropsicofarmacologia, Napoli 1967.

10 BUFALARI, A.: L'uso del trazodone in medicina interna. Clin. europ. *11:* 1–11 (1972).

11 BUOMPADRE, A.; MONTI, G. B. e ODERIO, A.: Studio del trazodone in preanestesia. Policlinico, Sez. med. *79:* 229–240 (1972).

12 BURBERI, P.; BURBERI, S., and SILVESTRINI, B.: Experimental toxicological tests with benzydamine. Boll. chim. farm. *108:* 781–788 (1969).

13 BURBERI, P.; PICCINELLI, D., and SILVESTRINI, B.: Effects of systematically administered drugs on intraocular pressure in rabbits. Arzneimittelforsch. *20:* 1143–1147 (1970).

14 CATANESE, B. and LISCIANI, R.: Investigations on the absorption and distribution of trazodone or AF 1161 in rats, dogs and humans. Boll. chim. farm. *109:* 369–373 (1970).

15 CEINO, A.: Clinical evaluation on the use of trittico (trazodone) in psychic disturbances in geriatric patients (in press).

16 CIANCHETTI, C. e GAINOTTI, G.: Studio clinico controllato dell'attività antidepressiva e ansiolitica di un nuovo psicofarmaco, l'AF 1161. Gazz. int. Med. Chir., Roma *73:* 1–10 (1968).

17 CIOFFI, F.; MATTIOLI, G.; POZZI, O. e RINALDI, F.: Ulteriori dati sull'azione antidepressiva di un nuovo psicofarmaco: l'AF 1161. Rass. int. Clin. Terap. *49:* 1483–1487 (1969).

18 CONTI, L.; PLACIDI, G. F.; BIAGINI, G. L.; MAGGINI, C. e CASTROGIOVANNI, P.: Studio clinico e poligrafico di un derivato del triazolo-4-3-alfa-piridina (AF 1161). Boll. Soc. Med. chir. Pisa *37:* 226–239 (1969).

19 COREA, L.: Trazodone in the treatment of anxiety occurring in internal medicine (in press).

20 COZZOLINO, G.; PAZZAGLIA, I.; DE GAETANO, V., and MACRI, M.: Clinical investigation on the possible interaction between anticoagulants and a new psychotropic drug (trazodone) (in press).

21 DANIELE, S. and FIORE, C.: Hypotensive effect on intra-ocular tension by AF 161 (trazodone). Ann. Oftal. *48:* 1–6 (1972).

22 DIONISIO, A.; SIGNORE, L. e DELOGU, G.: Considerazioni tossicologiche su di un nuovo psicoformaco: il trazodone. Rev. clin. Tossicol. *5–6:* 403–422 (1971).

23 DE FEO, G.; PICCINELLI, D. e SILVESTRINI, B.: Effetti di alcuni farmaci sulla motilità intestinale del topo normale e del topo trattato con tremorina. Farmaco *26:* 3–10 (1971).

24 GALVAN, L.; NAIR, N. P. V.; KUSSIN, D., and BAN, T. A.: Trazodone in the treatment of schizophrenias. Current Therapeutic Research *15:* 766–780 (1973).

25 GENTILI, E. e DIONISIO, A.: Informazioni cliniche sullo studio di un nuovo psicofarmaco: il trazodone (AF 1161). Riv. Neuropsichiat. *15:* 185–194 (1969).

26 GERARDI, A. U.: Indagine clinica preliminare del trazodone in preanestesia. Minerva Anest. (1973).

27 DI GIUSEPPE, B. e CESARINI, F.: Un nuovo psicofarmaco nella terapia delle depressioni. Clin. neuropsichiat. *5:* 3–11 (1965).

28 DI GIUSEPPE, B. e DIONISIO, A.: Un nuovo psicofarmaco, il 'trazodone', nella terapia delle psicosi cicloidi. Clin. neuropsichiat. *6:* 4–18 (1970).

29 DE GREGORIO, M.: Use of trazodone as a tranquilizer in routine medical practice: comparison with diazepam. Preliminary report (unpublished, 1971).

30 DE GREGORIO, M. e DIONISIO, A.: Ricerche cliniche su un nuovo psicofarmaco (AF 1161), valutazione preliminare. Med. psicosom. *14:* 477–493 (1969).

31 DE GREGORIO, M. and DIONISIO, A.: A controlled clinical study of a new antidepressant (trazodone). Panminerva med. *13:* 27–30 (1971).

32 GUNELLA, G. and MELICA, A.: Trazodone's effects on patients with partial or total ventilatory insufficiency (unpublished, 1973).

33 KNOBEL, M.: Trazodone and psychosomatic medicine. Proc. Round Table Discussion on Trazodone, 2nd Meet. Int. College of Psychosomatic Medicine, Amsterdam 1973.

34 MAGGINI, C.; GALLEVI, M.; CONTI, L.; PLACIDI, G. F. e CASTROGIOVANNI, P.: Impiego dell'indagine poligrafica del sonno nello studio delle caratteristiche terapeutiche di un nuovo psicofarmaco (AF 1161). Boll. Soc. med. chir., Pisa *37:* 294–305 (1969),

35 NAIR, N. P. V.; BAN, T. A.; HONTELA, S., and CLARKE, R.: Trazodone in the treatment of organic brain syndromes with special reference to psycho-geriatrics. Current Therapeutic Research *15:* 755–769 (1973).

36 PACIARONI, E.: Clinical report on the use of low doses of trazodone in geriatric patients (unpublished).

37 PALAZZO, G.: Chemistry of trazodone. Current Therapeutic Research *15:* 745–748 (1973).

38 PARIANTE, F.: Un nuovo antidepressivo: il trazodone – valutazione della sua attività con studio double-blind con cross-over. Riv. Neuropsichiat. *17:* 1–19 (1971).

39 PENNESI, S. O.: Nella terapia delle nevrosi: un nuovo psicofarmaco, il trittico. Riv. Neuropsichiat. *17:* 51–58 (1971).

40 POZZI, O.; MARGHERITA, G. e RINALDI, F.: Studio clinico doppio cieco cross-over sull'attività antidepressiva dell'AF 1161. Quad. Osped. psichiat. interprov. Salentino *2:* 250–258 (1967).

41 PRETOLANI, E.: Interesse di un nuovo psicofarmaco nelle malattie internistiche a componente psicosomatica. Clin. europ. *11:* 3–8 (1972).

42 REGGIANI, A.; MARTINI, G. e DIONISIO, A.: L'uso nell'endoscopia urologica di un nuovo psicofarmaco: il trazodone. Clin. europ. *11:* 293–309 (1972).

43 RUGGIERO, P;. BELLINI, G., and BRANDINELLI, E.: Our experiences with AF 1161 (trazodone) as a pre-anesthetic medication (in press).

44 SIGNORE, L.; ALTISSIMI, C.; MASTROSTEFANO, P. e MALIZIA, E.: Validità di un nuovo farmaco, l'AF 1161 o trazodone, nella preparazione del malato all'intervento chirurgico. Clin. ter. *57:* 155–162 (1971).

45 SILVESTRINI, B.: Pharmacological outline of a new psychodrug. Proc. 1st Nat. Meet. Italian Society of Neuropsychopharmacology, Naples 1967.

46 SILVESTRINI, B. and LISCIANI, R.: Pharmacology of trazodone. Current Therapeutic Research *15:* 749–754 (1973).

47 SILVESTRINI, B. and QUADRI, E.: Investigations on the specificity of the so-called analgesic activity of non-narcotic drugs. Europ. J. Pharmacol. *12:* 231–235 (1970).

48 TANSELLA, M. e DELLO RUSSO, G.: Il problema della valutazione pre-clinica dei nuovi farmaci psicotropi. Prime osservazioni cliniche sull'attività di un nuovo psicofarmaco (AF 1161). Acta neurol., Napoli *24:* 875–891 (1969).

49 UCHA UDABE, R.: Clinical experience with a new psychotropic drug – trazodone (a review of literature). Current Therpeutic Research *15:* 755–763 (1973).

50 VINAŘ, O.: Introductory remarks. Current Therapeutic Research *15:* 743–744 (1973).

51 VINCI, M.: Contributo clinico alla terapia delle depressioni endogene con un derivato delle triazolo-piridine. Osped. psichiat. *39:* 416–433 (1971).

52 VINCI, M. e IACOMETTA, T.: Considerazioni pratiche sugli effetti psichiatrici ed anestesici nella terapia elettroconvulsivante di un nuovo derivato del triazolo-4-3-alfa-piridina (trazodone). Osped. psichiat. (1973).

Author's address: Prof. J. SAARMA, Chief, Laboratory of Psychopharmacology, Department of Psychiatry, Tartu State University, *Tartu, Estonian SSR* (USSR).

Trazodone. Mod. Probl. Pharmacopsychiat., vol. 9, pp. 110–126,
ed. Th. A. Ban, Montreal, Que., and B. Silvestrini, Rome (Karger, Basel 1974)

Comprehensive Clinical Studies with Trazodone in Canada

THOMAS A. BAN, M. M. AMIN, N. P. V. NAIR and F. ENGELSMAN

Division of Psychopharmacology and Department of Psychiatry, McGill University, Montreal

Introduction to Canadian Studies

Chemical Aspects

Trazodone, a phenyl-piperazine derivative of triazolo-pyridine, was synthesized by PALAZZO in 1966. It consists of a triazolo-pyridine ring and a phenyl-piperazinyl-alkyl moiety (fig. 1). Although there are some other triazolo-pyridine substances patented with stimulant and tranquilizing properties, trazodone is the first triazolo-pyridine compound to be subjected to clinical psychopharmacological investigation.

Unlike the triazolo-pyridine nucleus, the phenyl-piperazinyl-alkyl moiety has been employed in clinical psychopharmacological studies and one phenyl-piperazinyl-alkyl preparation, oxypertine, has been shown to have psychotherapeutic properties, i. e. neuroleptic, antidepressant and anxiolytic effects.

Animal Pharmacological Data

On the basis of systematic animal pharmacological investigations, carried out by SILVESTRINI *et al.* [1968], it was suggested that trazodone may have psychotropic properties. As shown in table I, on two of seven variables (spontaneous motor activity and hexobarbital-induced sleeping time) trazodone produces nonspecific psycholeptic effects, and on two other variables (conditional avoidance reflex and amphetamine group toxicity) the action of the drug is similar to that of the neuroleptics. Unlike neuro-

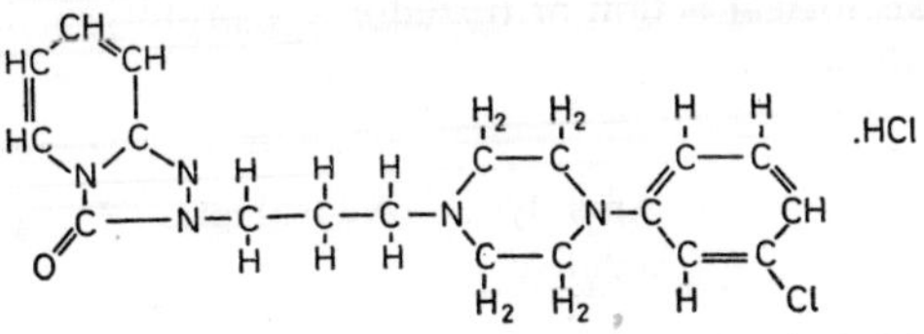

Fig. 1. Structural formula of trazodone.

leptics, however, trazodone does not decrease body temperature and does not have cataleptogenic effects. On the other hand, like some of the anxiolytic sedative drugs, it interferes with multineuronal reflexes. Nevertheless, since trazodone decreases the response to painful stimuli at doses lower than those which affect normal behavior, SILVESTRINI and LISCIANI [1973] speculate that trazodone may have a therapeutic effect in those conditions in which the emotional integration of unpleasant experiences play a role, e. g. depression.

Human Pharmacological Data

To supplement the animal pharmacological data, a psychometric study was carried out with five normal volunteers. Each experimental subject was given 25 mg of trazodone orally and was exposed to a battery of psychometric tests prior to and 2 h after drug administration. Testing time was chosen on the basis of the results of CATANESE and LISCIANI [1970] who found that maximal blood concentration of trazodone occurred in 120 min after oral drug administration [BAN *et al.*, 1973].

Results of the human pharmacological study are presented in table II. Needless to say, the experimental population included in this psychometric investigation was far too small for sophisticated statistical analysis. Nevertheless, the improvement in psychomotor test performance (auditory reaction time, tapping speed and track tracer time) suggests that trazodone may have psychoanaleptic, more specifically psychomotor-stimulating properties. In favor of a possible antidepressant action is the decrease in cancellation test error, suggesting improvement in concentration, associated with an increase in psychomotor speed. Since disintegration of mental faculties may be the result of impaired processing of sensory perceptual information, the finding that a lowered perceptual input (decreased critical flicker fusion

Table I. Comparative pharmacological action of trazodone, a prototype neuroleptic and a prototype anxiolytic-sedative

Variables	Anxiolytic sedative	Neuroleptic	Trazodone
Spontaneous motor activity	–	–	–
Hexobarbital-induced sleeping time	+	+	+
Conditional avoidance reflex	0	–	–
Amphetamine group toxicity	0	–	–
Body temperature	0	–	0
Cataleptogenic effect	0	+	0
Multi-neuronal reflexes	–	+	–

Table II. Changes in test performance of human volunteers under the influence of trazodone

Perceptual tests	Performance before (in means)	after (in means)	difference (in means)
Perceptual			
CFF	46.66	42.50	— 4.16
Psychomotor			
ART	169.40	155.00	—14.40
TAP	62.25	63.75	+ 1.50
TTT	86.20	76.40	— 9.80
Attention			
CTE	2.20	1.60	— 0.60

Critical flicker fusion frequency = CFF; auditory reaction time = ART; tapping speed = TAP; track tracer time = TTT; cancellation test error = CTE.

frequency) is associated with improvement in attention (concentration) and psychomotor function, raises the possibility that trazodone may be a therapeutically effective drug in the treatment of organic brain syndrome.

Methodology of Canadian Studies

Since findings in preliminary clinical trials substantiated the psychotropic effects of trazodone, but could not clearly define its actual therapeutic indications, a systematic clinical study was designed, including a total of 200 patients in 12 clinical drug trials. The first stage of this study was oriented to reveal the range of therapeutic activity of trazodone and entailed four independent clinical trials in four distinctly different psychiatric populations: organic brain syndrome, schizophrenia, depression and neurosis. To verify the therapeutic activity of trazodone in those patient groups where measurable beneficial changes occur under the influence of the investigational drug the uncontrolled clinical trials were planned to be supplemented with placebo-controlled clinical studies. Finally, in those patient groups in which therapeutic activity was verified, a series of standard-controlled clinical trials was planned to be undertaken in order to establish the comparative efficacy and differential therapeutic action of trazodone with regard to commonly employed psychoactive preparations.

Results of Canadian Studies

In this presentation results of the first five clinical trials are reported, and the differential findings with trazodone in the treatment of organic brain syndrome, schizophrenia and depression are discussed.

Organic Brain Syndrome

The experimental population of the first clinical drug trial carried out in organic brain syndrome patients consisted of 10 geriatric inpatients, seven females and three males, ranging in age from 65 to 84 years with a mean of 76 years (table III). All patients were diagnosed as suffering from organic brain syndrome and had a minimum score of one or two of the three items of the organic factor, i. e. memory disturbance, consciousness

Table III. Demographic data of the uncontrolled clinical trial in organic brain syndrome

Patient	Age, years	Sex	Diagnosis
1	66	M	senile dementia
2	78	M	senile dementia
3	72	M	senile dementia
4	74	F	psychosis with cerebral arteriosclerosis
5	79	F	psychosis with cerebral arteriosclerosis
6	74	F	senile dementia
7	80	F	senile dementia
8	78	F	senile dementia
9	85	F	senile dementia
10	83	F	senile dementia

alteration and dementia, on the Modified Verdun Target Symptom Rating Scale (VTSRS).

The clinical drug trial commenced with a 4-day placebo washout period. Drug administration followed a fixed changing dosage schedule, ranging from 25 to 125 mg per day, over a period of 84 days. Psychiatric assessments were based on interviews and observations carried out at regular intervals, on the basis of which the VTSRS, the Plutchik Geriatric Rating Scale (PGRS), the Brief Psychiatric Rating Scale (BPRS) and the Clinical Global Impression Scale (CGI) were scored. The VTSRS was also completed one week after discontinuation of trazodone administration.

As a result it was found that maximum improvement – maximal decrease in total VTSRS scores – was obtained on the dosage of 100 mg per day. Improvement in total VTSRS scores in the course of the clinical trial reached the accepted level of statistical significance ($p < 0.05$, analysis of covariance); and withdrawal of medication resulted in significant deterioration ($p < 0.05$, t-test) within one week. It was observed that increase in medication beyond 100 mg per day did not enhance therapeutic effects and may have even had a negative therapeutic effect (fig. 2). Further analysis of the VTSRS revealed that the most significant improvement occurred in the clusters of mood (depression) and organicity ($p < 0.01$). Findings on the PGRS and the BPRS were similar to that of the VTSRS. As shown in

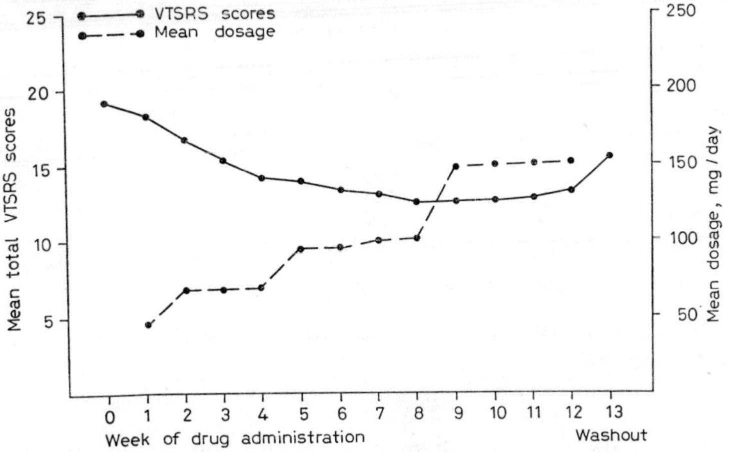

Fig. 2. Weekly changes in mean total Verdun Target Symptom Rating Scale scores in the course of the clinical drug trial.

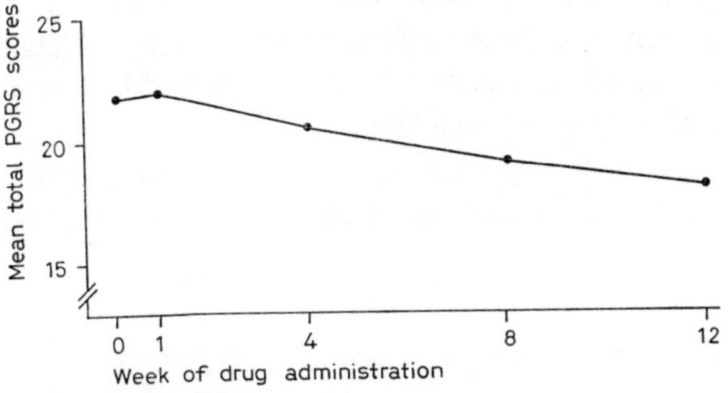

Fig. 3. Changes in mean total Plutchik Geriatric Rating Scale scores in the course of the clinical drug trial.

figure 3, there was a slight transient deterioration in the mean total scores of the PGRS, after one week of drug administration, which was followed by a steady improvement by the end of week four, eight and twelve; and as shown in figure 4, there was a slight but steady improvement (decrease) in the mean total scores of the BPRS. This was primarily due to a statistically significant improvement in motor retardation ($p < 0.05$) and to some improvement in depressive mood and anxiety. Finally at the end of the clinical drug trial, two patients were rated on the CGI as much improved, four as minimally improved and four as unchanged.

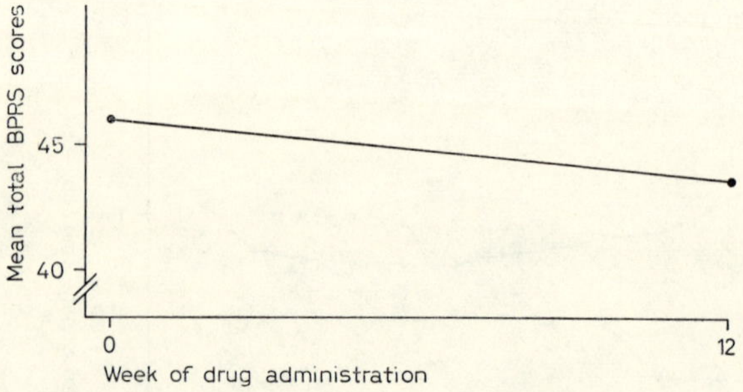

Fig. 4. Changes in mean total Brief Psychiatric Rating Scale scores in the course of the clinical drug trial.

There were six different adverse reactions reported in six patients during the clinical drug trial. The most frequent adverse reaction was excitement (four patients) and transient confusional state (two patients). It should be noted that one of the adverse effects, i. e. headache (migraine type) occurred in a patient 10 days after discontinuation of trazodone administration. This patient had been suffering from attacks of headache prior to the commencement of trazodone administration and had been free of this during the clinical drug trial (table IV).

To verify the beneficial therapeutic activity of trazodone in organic brain syndrome patients a placebo-controlled clinical trial is in progress.

Schizophrenia

The experimental population of the first clinical drug trial carried out in schizophrenic patients, consisted of ten chronic hospitalized patients, four females and six males, ranging in age from 48 to 57 years with a mean of 49.7 years. All patients were hospitalized longer than one year and had a minimum score of 27 on the BPRS.

The clinical drug trial commenced with a 14-day placebo washout period. Drug administration followed a fixed changing dosage schedule, ranging from 25 to 450 mg per day, over a period of 84 days. Psychiatric assessments were based on interviews and observations carried out at regular intervals on the basis of which the BPRS and CGI were scored. The BPRS was also completed one week after discontinuation of trazodone administration.

Table IV. Adverse effects reported during the uncontrolled clinical trial in organic brain syndrome patients

Adverse Effects	Number of patients with symptoms
I Psychiatric	
Confusional state	2
Drowsiness	1
Excitement	4
Insomnia	1
II Neurological	
Headache	1
III Autonomic	
Diarrhea	1

As a result it was found that maximum improvement – maximal decrease in total BPRS scores – was obtained on the dosage of 300 mg per day. There was a slight decrease (improvement) in total BPRS scores by the end of the fourth week of treatment, followed by a fluctuating increase of psychopathology for the remaining period of drug administration. Withdrawal of medication, however, resulted in further deterioration. It was observed that increase in medication beyond 300 mg per day did not enhance therapeutic effects and may even have had a negative therapeutic effect (fig. 5). While at no time did the change in total BPRS scores reach the accepted level of statistical significance ($p < 0.05$), further analysis of the BPRS revealed that the greatest improvement of the BPRS items was seen in somatic concern and depressive mood and the greatest deterioration in grandiosity and hallucinatory behavior. Finally, at the end of the clinical drug trial, one patient was rated on the CGI as very much improved, three as minimally improved, four as minimally worse and two as much worse.

Adverse reactions were encountered in all but one patient, with the number of adverse reactions per patient ranging from one (in four patients) to three (in three patients). It should be noted that in one patient drug administration was transiently discontinued for 12 days because of hypertension (250/120 Hg nm) associated with atrial arrhythmia. Both adverse effects spontaneously remitted and did not recur upon resumption of administration of the investigational drug (table V).

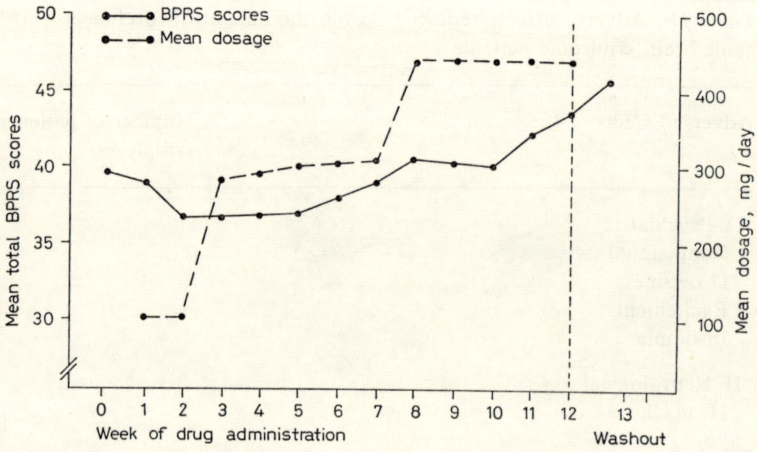

Fig. 5. Weekly changes in mean total Brief Psychiatric Rating Scale scores in the course of the clinical drug trial.

Table V. Adverse effects reported during the uncontrolled clinical trial in schizophrenic patients

Adverse Effects	Number of patients with symptoms
I Psychiatric	
Agitation	1
Anxiety	1
Asthenia	1
Insomnia	1
Tension	1
II Autonomic	
Atrial arrythmia	1
Dry mouth	1
Hypertension	1
III Miscellaneous	
Abnormal hematology	2
Abnormal liver function	1
Headache	2
Weight gain	1

Table VI. Percentage of patients with improvement, no change and deterioration with trazodone and with an inactive placebo (BPRS)

Drug	Deterioration, %	No change, %	Improvement, %
Trazodone	35	40	25
Placebo	50	40	10

The uncontrolled clinical trial in chronic schizophrenic patients was supplemented with a placebo-controlled clinical study including a total of 20 experimental subjects. Analysis of data from the placebo-controlled clinical trial is in progress. Nevertheless, by pooling the data from the two completed studies, table VI shows that a lower percentage of patients deteriorated and a higher percentage of patients improved with trazodone than with an inactive placebo.

Depression

The experimental population of the first clinical drug trial carried out in depressed patients consisted of ten psychiatric patients, nine females and one male, ranging in age from 24 to 46 years with a mean of 34.7 years. All patients were diagnosed as suffering from depression – seven reactive and three endogenous – and had a minimum score of 25 on the Hamilton Depression Rating Scale (HAM) at the time of the initial assessment.

The clinical drug trial commenced with a 7-day placebo washout period. Drug administration followed a fixed changing dosage schedule, ranging from 25 to 300 mg per day, over a period of 56 days. Psychiatric assessments were based on interviews and observations carried out at regular intervals, on the basis of which the HAM, BPRS and CGI were scored. The HAM was also completed one week after discontinuation of trazodone administration.

As a result it was found that maximum improvement – maximal decrease in total HAM scores – was obtained in the dosage of 75 mg per day. The decrease (improvement) in total HAM scores reached the accepted level of statistical significance ($p < 0.001$, analysis of variance). With-

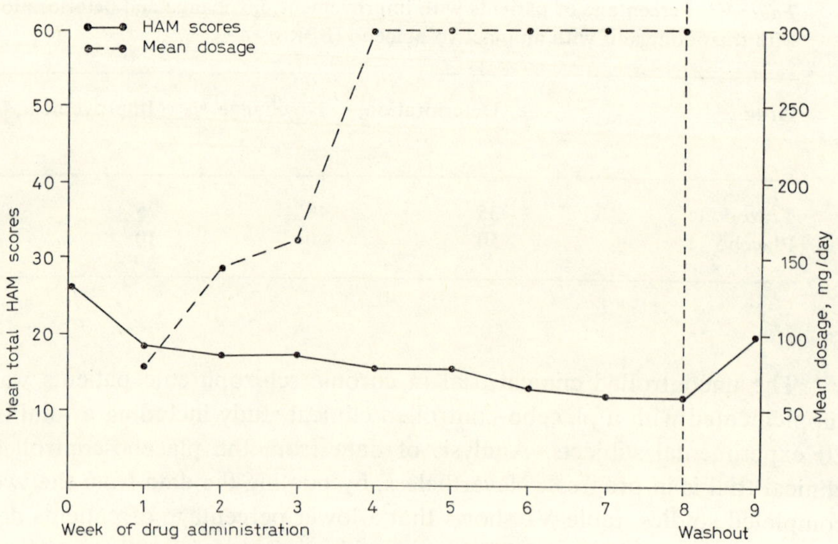

Fig. 6. Weekly changes in mean total Hamilton Psychiatric Rating Scale for Depression scores in the course of the clinical drug trial.

drawal of medication resulted in clinical deterioration, i. e. an increase in total scores. It was observed that increase in medication beyond 75 mg per day did not appreciably increase therapeutic effects (fig. 6). Further analysis – employing analysis of covariance – indicated a significant ($p < 0.01$) change in three factors of the HAM, i. e. anxiety-depression, sleep disturbance and apathy. Findings on the BPRS were similar to that of the HAM. There was a significant ($p < 0.05$) decrease (improvement) of scores in four items, i. e. anxiety, guilt feeling, tension and suspiciousness. Finally, at the end of the clinical drug trial five patients were rated as much improved, three as minimally improved, one as unchanged and one as minimally worse.

Adverse reactions were encountered in all patients, with the number of adverse reactions per patient ranging from three to eleven. It was noted that 92% of all adverse reactions had been reported by the end of week four and with dosages above the optimal therapeutic dosage of trazodone (table VII). One of the patients found her 'tremor' similar to that under the influence of chlorpromazine. Nevertheless, while the chlorpromazine-in-

Table VII. Adverse effects reported during the uncontrolled clinical trial in depressed patients

Adverse Effects	Number of patients with symptoms
I Psychiatric	
Aggressiveness	1
Drowsiness	2
Excitement	2
Increased libido	1
Insomnia	1
Toxic confusional state	2
II Neurological	
Akathisia	1
Blurred vision	2
Dizziness	1
Tremor	4
III Autonomic	
Constipation	3
Diarrhea	1
Dry mouth	6
Hypotension	2
Sweating	1
Tachycardia	3
IV Miscellaneous	
Headache	4
Nausea	2

Table VIII. Percentage of patients with improvement, no change and deterioration with trazodone and with amitriptyline (HAM)

Drug	Deterioration, %	No change, %	Improvement, %
Trazodone	10	10	80
Amitriptyline	10	20	70

Table IX. The eight items of the HAM in which statistically significant improvement occurred with trazodone

Items	F	p
Anxiety Psychic	2.6	0.01
Somatic symptoms, gastrointestinal	2.2	0.05
Loss of weight	5.3	0.01
Feelings of guilt	2.7	0.01
Depressed mood	3.9	0.01
Early insomnia	2.6	0.01
Paranoid symptoms	2.4	0.05
Obsessional and compulsive symptoms	1.9	0.05

duced tremor responded to trihexyphenidyl (Artane), the trazodone-induced tremor did not. On the other hand, the trazodone-induced tremor did respond to diphenhydramine (Benadryl). Subsequently, diphenhydramine was successfully employed in three cases with tremors and also in one patient for the control of excitement.

To verify the beneficial therapeutic activity of trazodone in depressed patients a placebo-controlled clinical trial is in progress; and in order to establish the comparative efficacy and differential therapeutic action of trazodone with regard to amitriptyline, a commonly employed tricyclic antidepressant, a standard-controlled clinical trial, including a total of 20 experimental subjects has been carried out. Analysis of data of the standard-controlled clinical trial is in progress. Nevertheless, by pooling the data from the two completed clinical studies, table VIII shows that a lower percentage of patients remained unchanged and a higher percentage of patients improved with trazodone than with amitriptyline. Furthermore, an analysis of variance (repeated measures model) yielded significant F ratios in the total scores as well as on eight items of the HAM, i. e. depressed mood, anxiety psychic, somatic symptoms, gastrointestinal, loss of weight, feelings of guilt, early insomnia, paranoid symptoms and obsessional and compulsive symptoms (table IX). As shown in figure 7, overall improvement was more rapid with trazodone than with amitriptyline and as shown in figure 8, 9 and 10 it was also more smooth. Trazodone produced somewhat lower incidence of adverse effects.

Table X. The most characteristic trazodone responsive psychopathological symptoms in the three different groups

Organic brain syndrome	Schizophrenia	Depression
Depressive mood	(depressive mood)	depressive mood
Motor retardation	(somatic concern)	anxiety psychic
Organicity		paranoid symptoms

Parentheses indicate lack of statistical significance.

Place of Trazodone in Contemporary Therapy

The most characteristic findings with trazodone, in the three different diagnostic groups studied, are presented in table X. These results strongly suggest that trazodone has a therapeutic effect in psychiatric patients suffering from depression. It is well established, that 30–40 % of depressed patients show a favorable therapeutic response to an inactive placebo and that 60–70 % improve on commercially available dibenzazepine (e. g. imipramine) and dibenzocycloheptene (e. g. amitriptyline) drugs. In view of this, if the 80-percent improvement rate of the Canadian studies could be confirmed, trazodone would be in a favorable position among the antidepressants.

Therapeutic responsiveness to trazodone cut across the traditional nosological categories; it also cuts across the clinical syndromes which are affected by monoamine oxidase inhibitors or tricyclic antidepressants. Furthermore, since therapeutic responsiveness to trazodone includes positive changes in depressive mood, psychic anxiety and paranoid symptoms without negative therapeutic effects in schizophrenia, trazodone may become particularly useful in the treatment of depression in schizophrenia and in the treatment of involutional syndrome regardless whether it is diagnosed as involutional melancholia or involutional paranoia. Finally, if our findings – potent therapeutic action with low incidence of adverse effects – in organic brain syndrome could be substantiated, trazodone would become an important tool in the treatment of psychogeriatric patients.

Needless to say, to date there is no sufficient evidence to substantiate all of these therapeutic claims. On the other hand, on the basis of the

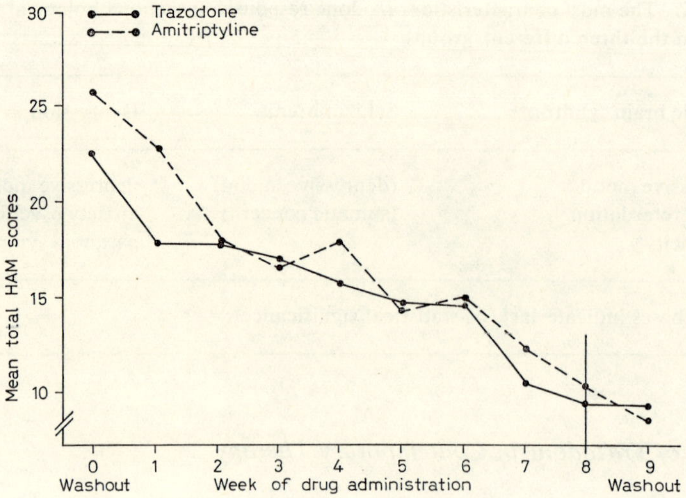

Fig. 7. Weekly changes in the mean total Hamilton Psychiatric Rating Scale for Depression scores with trazodone and amitriptyline in the course of the clinical drug trial.

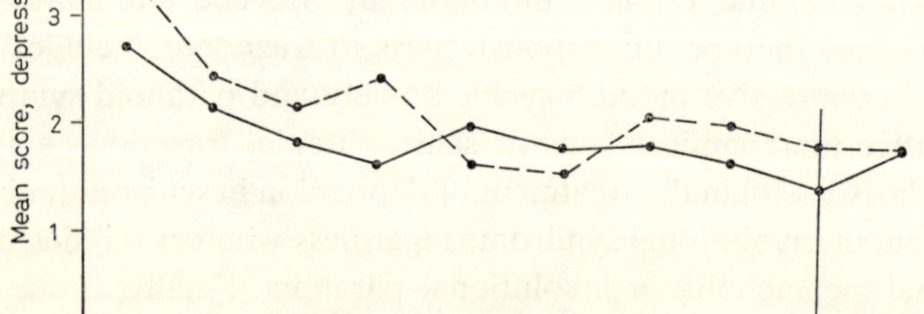

Fig. 8. Weekly changes in the mean scores of the item Depressed Mood on the Hamilton Psychiatric Rating Scale for Depression.

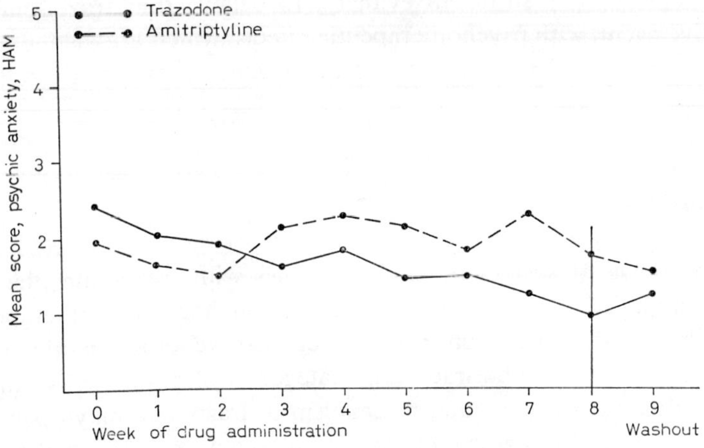

Fig. 9. Weekly changes in the mean scores of the item Anxiety Psychic on the Hamilton Psychiatric Rating Scale for Depression.

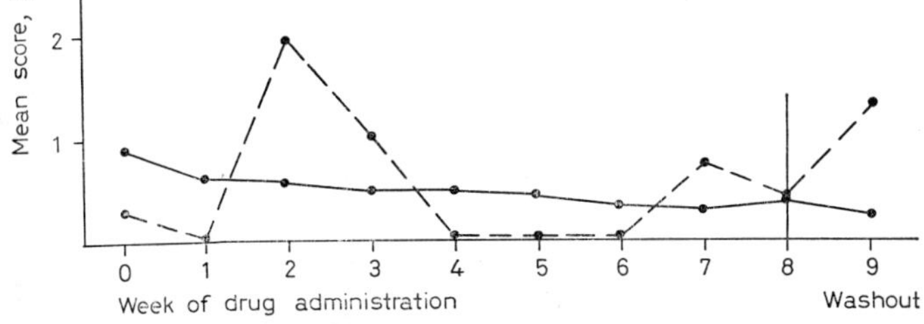

Fig. 10. Weekly changes in the mean scores of the item Paranoid Symptoms on the Hamilton Psychiatric Rating Scale for Depression.

Canadian data there is sufficient evidence to believe that trazodone is a psychoactive agent, with psychotherapeutic effects, which are distinctly different from traditional neuroleptic, antidepressant or anxiolytic sedative drugs.

Conclusions

In the course of systematic clinical studies with trazodone, the first clinically employed triazolo-pyridine preparation, the psychotherapeutic effects of the new drug were confirmed. Since the psychotherapeutic profile of trazodone cuts across the traditional categories of psychoactive drugs, further clarification of the action mechanism of trazodone may open new avenues in our understanding of psychopathology and the psychiatric patient.

References

BAN, T. A.; LEHMANN, H. E.; AMIN, M. M.; GALVAN, L.; NAIR, N. P. V.; VERGARA, L., and ZOCH, C.: Comprehensive clinical studies with trazodone. Curr. ther. Res. *15:* 540–551 (1973).

CATANESE, B. and LISCIANI, R.: Investigation of the absorption and distribution of trazodone or AF 1161 in rats, dogs and humans. Boll. chim. farm. *109:* 369–373 (1970).

PALAZZO, G. (1966): in ACRAF Product Monogr. on trazodone, Montreal 1972.

SILVESTRINI, B.; CIOLI, V.; BURBERI, S., and CATANESE, B.: Pharmacological properties of AF 1161, a new psychotropic drug. Int. J. Neuropharmacol. *7:* 587–599 (1968).

SILVESTRINI, B. and LISCIANI, R.: Pharmacology of trazodone (in press, 1973).

Author's address: Dr. T. A. BAN, Division of Psychopharmacology, Department of Psychiatry, McGill University, *Montreal* (Canada)

Trazodone. Mod. Probl. Pharmacopsychiat., vol. 9, pp. 127–139,
ed. Th. A. Ban, Montreal, Que., and B. Silvestrini, Rome (Karger, Basel 1974)

Trazodone in the Treatment of Neurosis

F. ANTONELLI, M. DE GREGORIO, A. DIONISIO and D. PERUZY
Research Department of the Italian Society of Psychosomatic Medicine, Rome

Trazodone in the Treatment of Neuroses

The therapeutic effectiveness of trazodone in patients with neurotic disorders has been proved in controlled clinical trials carried out in recent years [GRIECO, 1971; OLIVIERI-PENNESI, 1971; ARGENTA, 1972]. It has been found that trazodone is active in neurotic patients at daily doses ranging from 75 to 150 mg, that it has an effect which can be detected as early as the 7th day of treatment, and that it is capable of influencing the following symptoms in particular: anxiety, tension, somatic symptoms and concerns, loss of interest, insomnia, lowering of mood-tone and psychomotor retardation.

A clinical investigation in the field of psychoneurosis was planned in order to widen the knowledge of the therapeutic range of this new psychotropic drug.

In a preliminary double-blind placebo-controlled trial [ANTONELLI *et al.*, 1973] our findings substantiated the observations made by the other authors.

The present double-blind standard-controlled study was undertaken to determine which type of psychoneurosis showed the greatest response to trazodone.

Experimental Method and Procedure

A total of 168 psychoneurotic out-patients were admitted to the trial, provided that the selection criteria listed below were met: (1) subjects ranging in age from 18 to 70 years; (2) no history, or suspicion of concurrent psychosis; (3) diagnosis of anxiety reaction, mixed anxiety-depressive reaction, obsessive reaction (with contemporaneous presence of phobias, obsessions and compulsions), conversion reaction.

Pregnant women and patients with a recent or concurrent organic illness were excluded from the study. The patients were subdivided into groups according to the above-mentioned diagnoses.

After a 7-day placebo washout period, patients of each diagnostic group were randomly assigned to the treatment sub-groups (trazodone, diazepam and placebo sub-groups).

At the end of the study, the selected patients with the diagnosis of conversion reaction were only ten and the relevant treatment sub-groups were unbalanced. For this reason, the data pertaining to those patients were not considered in the analysis of the results.

The experimental population ($n = 158$) is described in table I. It can be calculated from table I that there was no statistical difference between treatment groups with regard to sex distribution ($p > 0.50$), mean age ($p > 0.50$) and diagnosis ($p > 0.50$).

Trazodone 25 mg, diazepam 5 mg and placebo were supplied in matching capsules and packaged in separate bottles, identified by code numbers, for each patient. Each bottle contained 42 capsules. The patients were treated for two weeks at the fixed dosage of 1 capsule t. i. d. under double-blind conditions. The same dosage schedule was also used for the placebo, administered during the washout period. During the trial no concomitant therapy was administered.

Assessment of therapeutic efficacy was based on the following criteria:

1. Global clinical rating was done on a four-point scale on each patient at the end of the experimental treatment. The therapeutic result was considered 'poor' if no improvement or deterioration occurred; 'fair' if there was a slight improvement; 'good' if decisive improvement occurred; 'excellent' if there was a complete or an almost complete remission of symptoms.

2. Wittenborn psychiatric rating scale (WPRS) was completed at the following times: time 0 = at the end of the washout period, i. e. immediately before the beginning of the experimental treatment; time 1 = on the 7th day of experimental treatment; time 2 = on the 14th day, i. e. at the end of the experimental treatment.

At the end of the experimental treatment period all the patients were questioned for the occurrence of side-effects.

Table I. Description of experimental population (n = 158)

Variables	Trazodone	Diazepam	Placebo
Number	54	50	54
Sex			
Males	26	27	31
Females	28	23	23
Age, years			
Range	21–68	18–66	19–68
Mean	40.4	41.5	41.6
Psychiatric diagnosis			
Anxiety reaction	18	19	14
Mixed anxiety-depressive reaction	25	24	28
Obsessive reaction	11	7	12

The G test[1] was used for the statistical elaboration of the qualitative data pertaining to the global clinical rating of improvement. In order to compare the effect of the three experimental treatments according to the WPRS, both the total score of the rating scale, as well as the score relative to each of the 6 symptom clusters were taken into consideration at the three above-mentioned times.

Within each diagnostic group following the control of the homogeneity of data at time 0 – according to the variance analysis – the statistical elaboration of data was carried out by means of the covariance analysis (i. e. both the values of time 1 as well as those of time 2 were adjusted to the pretreatment values).

In all the patients in whom a significant difference between treatments was observed, non-orthogonal paired comparisons were carried out by means of the F test using the adjusted values. In addition, a non-parametric method was used.

Within each diagnostic group following the control of the homogeneity of baseline data by means of the Kruskal-Wallis Test, the Mann-Whitney analysis was done on both the differences between values of time 0 and time 1 and the differences between values of time 0 and time 2.

1 Non-parametric test whose theoretical values are distributed as X^2 with the same number of degrees of freedom [WOOLF, 1957].

Table II. Double-blind study in psychoneurotic outpatients. Frequency distribution of the patients (n = 158) according to the treatment and the clinical result

Treatment	Therapeutic result				Total cases
	poor	fair	good	excellent	
Trazodone	7	6	24	17	54
Diazepam	11	13	17	9	50
Placebo	24	17	11	2	54

$\chi^2_{(6)}$ General = G = 34.79 ($p < 0.001$).
$\chi^2_{(3)}$ Trazodone versus diazepam = G = 7.09 (n. s.).
$\chi^2_{(3)}$ Drugs versus placebo = G = 27.70 ($p < 0.001$).
$\chi^2_{(3)}$ Trazodone versus placebo = G = 33.84 ($p < 0.001$).
$\chi^2_{(3)}$ Diazepam versus placebo = G = 11.44 ($p < 0.01$).

Results

Global Clinical Rating

The frequency distribution of the 158 psychoneurotic patients according to treatment and overall therapeutic response, as evaluated after 2 weeks of treatment in each patient, is reported in table II.

When these pooled results were analysed, both trazodone and diazepam were found superior to placebo (respectively $p < 0.001$ and $p < 0.01$). The improvement rate of the trazodone group was higher than that of the diazepam group, but the difference was not statistically significant. Analysis of the global clinical ratings assessed in psychoneurotic patients with the diagnosis of anxiety reaction is presented in table III. Trazodone and diazepam produced a therapeutic response in a similar number of patients.

Both drugs gave significantly better results than placebo ($p < 0.05$). The proportion of psychoneurotic patients with the diagnosis of mixed anxiety-depressive reaction responding to each treatment can be seen in table IV. Statistical analysis of these results indicated that both trazodone and diazepam were superior to placebo (respectively $p < 0.001$ and $p < 0.05$).

There was a clear trend towards better results in the trazodone sub-

Table III. Anxiety reaction. Frequency distribution of the patients (n = 51) according to the treatment and the clinical result

Treatment	Therapeutic result				Total cases
	poor	fair	good	excellent	
Trazodone	3	1	7	7	18
Diazepam	3	5	4	7	19
Placebo	8	2	3	1	14

$\chi^2_{(6)}$ General = G = 13.64 ($p < 0.05$).
$\chi^2_{(3)}$ Trazodone versus diazepam = G = 3.71 (n. s.).
$\chi^2_{(3)}$ Drugs versus placebo = G = 9.93 ($p < 0.05$).
$\chi^2_{(3)}$ Trazodone versus placebo = G = 8.90 ($p < 0.05$).
$\chi^2_{(3)}$ Diazepam versus placebo = G = 8.13 ($p < 0.05$).

Table IV. Mixed anxiety-depressive reaction. Frequency distribution of the patients (n = 77) according to the treatment and the clinical result

Treatment	Therapeutic result				Total cases
	poor	fair	good	excellent	
Trazodone	3	4	10	8	25
Diazepam	6	6	11	1	24
Placebo	13	11	3	1	28

$\chi^2_{(6)}$ General = G = 25.17 ($p < 0.001$).
$\chi^2_{(3)}$ Trazodone versus diazepam = G = 7.64 (n. s.).
$\chi^2_{(3)}$ Drugs versus placebo = G = 17.53 ($p < 0.001$).
$\chi^2_{(3)}$ Trazodone versus placebo = G = 20.13 ($p < 0.001$).
$\chi^2_{(3)}$ Diazepam versus placebo = G = 8.68 ($p < 0.05$).

group than in the diazepam sub-group (observed value of G test = 7.64, very close to theoretical value for the 5-percent level = 7.82).

It is evident from table V that no significant difference between treatments (trazodone, diazepam and placebo) was detected in patients with the diagnosis of 'obsessive reaction'.

Table V. Obsessive reaction. Frequency distribution of the patients (= 30) according to the treatment and the clinical result

Treatment	Therapeutic result				Total cases
	poor	fair	good	excellent	
Trazodone	1	1	7	2	11
Diazepam	2	2	2	1	7
Placebo	3	4	5	0	12

$\chi^2(6) = G = 7.31$ (n. s.).

Wittenborn Psychiatric Rating Scale

Analysis of variance of the baseline data is shown in table VI. A significant difference in the initial level of psychopathology among the three treatment sub-groups was observed only in the 'anxiety reaction' diagnostic group regarding factor IV (depressive retardation). Analysis of the baseline data referring to factor III (obsessive-compulsive-phobic) in the 'anxiety-reaction' diagnostic group and factor VI (paranoia) in all the diagnostic groups was not performed because the number of patients with the relevant symptoms was too small.

Similar considerations could be made about the Kruskal Wallis analysis of the baseline data (table VII).

Anxiety Reaction

Covariance analysis of WPRS scores after 1 week of treatment indicated no difference between treatments in the 'total score' and in all the symptom clusters apart from 'anxiety'. According to this parameter both trazodone and diazepam were superior to placebo ($p < 0.05$).

Covariance analysis of WPRS scores at time 2 is presented in table VIII which also shows that at the end of the second week of treatment the comparison between trazodone and placebo, as well as the comparison between diazepam and placebo, became statistically significant according to the total score and to the 'anxiety' and 'excitement' factors. No significant difference

Table VI. Variance analysis of WPRS scores at time 0 (before treatment)

WPRS scores	Anxiety reaction			Mixed anxiety-depressive reaction			Obsessive-compulsive reaction		
	d. f.		F	d. f.		F	d. f.		F
	n_1	n_2		n_1	n_2		n_1	n_2	
Total score	2	48	1.35	2	74	0.64	2	27	0.13
I. Anxiety	2	48	1.36	2	74	0.52	2	27	0.46
II. Somatic-hysterical	2	36	0.85	2	55	2.12	2	22	0.24
III. Obsessive-compulsive-phobic	–[1]	–	–	2	12	0.67	2	27	0.13
IV. Depressive retardation	2	39	6.40[2]	2	74	0.27	2	26	0.47
V. Excitement	2	40	0.29	2	45	2.35	2	19	0.39
VI. Paranoia	–	–	–	–	–	–	–	–	–

1 Analysis not performed since the number of patients with this symptom was too small.
2 Significant at 1 % level.

Table VII. Kruskal-Wallis analysis of WPRS scores at time 0 (before treatment)

WPRS scores	Anxiety reaction	Mixed anxiety-depressive reaction	Obsessive-compulsive reaction
Total score	3.11	3.92	3.65
I. Anxiety	2.90	0.47	0.58
II. Somatic-hysterical	0.36	1.61	0.40
III. Obsessive-compulsive-phobic	–[1]	0.05	0.17
IV. Depressive retardation	8.05[2,3]	0.36	1.48
V. Excitement	0.44	3.25	1.07
VI. Paranoia	–	–	–

1 Analysis not performed since the number of patients with this symptom was too small.
2 Significant at 5 % level.
3 Among the paired comparisons performed using the Mann-Whitney test only that relevant to 'diazepam versus placebo' showed to be not significant.

Table VIII. Anxiety reaction. Analysis of WPRS scores after 2 weeks of treatment

WPRS scores	Covariance analysis			Adjusted means[1]			Non-orthogonal comparisons of adjusted values				
	d. f.		F	placebo	diazepam	trazodone	d. f.		placebo vs. diazepam	placebo vs. trazodone	diazepam vs. trazodone
	n_1	n_2					n_1	n_2			
Total score	2	47	4.53[2]	7.92	4.83	5.19	1	47	7.82[3]	6.15[2]	0.11
I. Anxiety	2	47	6.03[3]	4.22	2.33	2.86	1	47	9.50[3]	4.84[2]	0.90
II. Somatic-hysterical	2	35	1.72	1.33	0.98	0.99					
V. Excitement	2	39	8.88[4]	1.77	0.73	0.85	1	39	18.33[4]	14.00[4]	0.20

1 Lower score indicates more improvement.
2 Significant at 5 % level.
3 Significant at 1 % level.
4 Significant at 0.1 % level.

Table IX. Anxiety reaction. WPRS scores after 2 weeks of treatment. Paired comparisons of the effect of the experimental treatments by means of the Mann-Whitney test[1]

WPRS scores	Placebo vs. diazepam	Placebo vs. trazodone	Diazepam vs. trazodone
Total score	–2.34[2]	–.2.68[3]	1.02
I. Anxiety	–2.66[3]	–2.09[2]	1.26
II. Somatic-hysterical	(–)	(–)	–1.07
IV. Depressive retardation	1.39		
V. Excitement	(–)[3]	(–)	0.83

1 Positive values of the Mann-Whitney test mean difference in favour of the first product. Negative values mean difference in favour of the second product. The symbols are in brackets in instances of N_A and/or $N_B < 10$.
2 Significant at 5% level.
3 Significant at 1% level.

between trazodone and diazepam was detected, although adjusted means indicated a trend towards greater improvement with diazepam.

The non-parametric analysis carried out by means of the Mann-Whitney test (table IX) confirmed the above-mentioned results.

Mixed Anxiety-Depressive Reaction

Time 1 results submitted to covariance analysis indicated an overall significant difference between treatments in 'total score' ($p < 0.05$) and in the 'somatic-hysterical' symptom cluster ($p < 0.01$). Trazodone was superior to placebo according to both the 'total score' ($p < 0.05$) and the 'somatic-hysterical' factor ($p < 0.001$). No significant difference was reached between diazepam and placebo. Similar results were obtained by means of the Mann-Whitney test on time 1 data. Covariance analysis of WPRS scores at time 2 (two weeks of treatment) is reported in table X.

The sub-group treated with trazodone improved to a greater extent than both the diazepam sub-group and the placebo sub-group, according to the 'total score' and to the 'anxiety', 'somatic-hysterical' and 'depressive retardation' factors.

Table X. Mixed anxiety-depressive reaction. Analysis of WPRS scores after 2weeks of treatment

WPRS scores	Covariance analysis d. f.			Adjusted means[1]			Non-orthogonal comparisons of adjusted values d. f.				
	n_1	n_2	F	placebo	diazepam	trazodone	n_1	n_2	placebo vs. diazepam	placebo vs. trazodone	diazepam vs. trazodone
Total score	2	73	5.58[2]	10.74	10.19	6.93	1	73	0.21	10.74[2]	6.94[3]
I. Anxiety	2	73	5.72[2]	5.00	4.64	3.06	1	73	0.36	11.39[2]	6.55[3]
II. Somatic-hysterical	2	54	3.31[3]	1.57	1.45	0.90	1	54	0.16	7.66[2]	4.42[3]
III. Obsessive-compulsive-phobic	2	11	0.35	2.20	3.06	2.11					
IV. Depressive retardation	2	73	28.95[4]	3.22	2.90	2.14	1	73	10.00[2]	116.00[4]	28.50[4]
V. Excitement	2	44	0.58	1.41	1.38	1.10					

1 Lower score indicates more improvement.
2 Significant at 1 % level.
3 Significant at 5 % level.
4 Significant at 0.1 % level.

Table XI. Mixed anxiety-depressive reaction. WPRS scores after 2 weeks of treatment. Paired comparisons of the effect of the experimental treatments by means of the Mann-Whitney test[1]

WPRS scores	Placebo vs. diazepam	Placebo vs. trazodone	diazepam vs. trazodone
Total score	−0.23	−.2.71[2]	−2.82[2]
I. Anxiety	−0.51	−2.73[2]	−2.14[3]
II. Somatic-hysterical	−0.53	−3.39[4]	−4.29[4]
III. Obsessive-compulsive-phobic	(+)	(±)	(−)
IV. Depressive retardation	−1.18	−2.74[2]	−1.74
V. Excitement	0.00	−0.43	−1.24

1 Positive values of the Mann-Whitney test mean difference in favour of the first product. Negative values mean difference in favour of the second product. The symbols are in brackets in instances of N_A and/or $N_B < 10$.
2 Significant at 1 % level.
3 Significant at 5 % level.
4 Significant at 0.1 % level.

Table XII. Side-effects reported according to treatment

Side-effect	Treatment		
	trazodone	diazepam	placebo
Drowsiness	4	5	1
Weakness	4	6	2
Insomnia	0	0	1
Restlessness	0	0	1
Dizziness	0	2	0
Blurred vision	0	1	0
Headache	0	0	1
Dry mouth	1	1	0
Increased sweating	1	0	0
Gastric complaints	3	1	0
Constipation	0	0	1
Patients with side-effects	10	11	6
Treated patients	54	50	54

There was a trend towards a greater improvement in the diazepam sub-group than in the placebo sub-group, but no significant difference could be detected. The non-parametric analysis of the 2-week treatment data confirmed the above-mentioned inferences (table XI).

Obsessive Reaction

Trazodone and diazepam were not demonstrably superior to placebo in patients with the diagnosis of 'obsessive reaction'. In fact, no significant difference between the three types of treatment could be detected in either the 'total score' or in any of the symptom clusters.

Side-Effects

Side-effects were reported in 10 of the 54 patients who received trazodone, 11 of the 50 patients who received diazepam and six of the 54 patients who received placebo.

Three patients in the trazodone group, five in the diazepam group and one in the placebo group complained of more than one side-effect. Table XII lists the side-effects in each treatment group. The side-effects reported were mild to moderate in severity, transient in nature, diminished in intensity or completely remitted with time and did not constitute a serious problem in therapy in any patient.

In both the trazodone group and the diazepam group the most frequently reported side-effects were drowsiness and weakness, which occurred during the first week of treatment.

Conclusions

In psychoneurotic patients with the diagnosis of 'anxiety reaction' both trazodone and diazepam produced a similar significant improvement in the 'anxiety' symptom cluster of WPRS after 1 week of treatment. After 2 weeks of treatment a tendency towards lower WPRS scores was seen in the diazepam treated sub-group, although no significant difference between the two drugs was obtained on analysis of both the 'global clinical ratings' and the 'WPRS' scores.

In the psychoneurotic patients with the diagnosis of 'mixed anxiety depressive reaction' trazodone produced a significantly greater improvement than diazepam in both the total score and the 'somatic-hysterical' factor of WPRS, after 1 week of treatment.

After 2 weeks of treatment a significant difference in favour of trazodone was detected in the 'anxiety' and 'depressive retardation' factors as well. Moreover, the trazodone sub-group tended to show better global clinical ratings than the diazepam sub-group.

In psychoneurotic patients with the diagnosis of 'obsessive reaction' neither trazodone nor diazepam differed significantly from placebo.

References

Antonelli, F.; De Gregorio, M., and Dionisio, A.: Trazodone in the treatment of psychoneuroses: a double-blind study. Curr. ther. Res. *15:* 799–804 (October supplement, 1973).

Argenta, G.: Il Trittico (trazodone) nella terapia dell'ansia. Policlinico, Sez. Med. *79:* 174–180 (1972).

Grieco, F.: Estudio clínico del trazodone. Proc. 1st Congr. Int. College of Psychosomatic Medicine, Guadalajara 1971.

Olivieri Pennesi, S.: Nella terapia delle nevrosi: un nuovo psicofarmaco, il trittico. Riv. Neuropsichiat. *17:* 51–58 (1971).

Woolf, B.: The log likelihood ratio test (the G test). Ann. hum. Genet. *21:* 397–409 (1957).

Author's address: Prof. Ferruccio Antonelli, Direttore della Cattedra di Medicina Psicosomatica dell'Università Cattolica di Roma, Viale della Camilluccia, 195, *I-00135 Roma* (Italy)

Trazodone. Mod. Probl. Pharmacopsychiat., vol. 9, pp. 140–145,
ed. Th. A. Ban, Montreal, Que., and B. Silvestrini, Rome (Karger, Basel 1974)

Preliminary Clinical Studies with Trazodone in the Treatment of Neurotic Patients

Sadanori Miura
School of Medicine, Kitasato University, Sagamihara

In recent years the tranquilizing effect of trazodone has been demonstrated by several workers. This presentation, part of an investigation on the anti-anxiety properties of trazodone, is based on the findings obtained in a preliminary open clinical trial carried out prior to a double-blind controlled study.

Method

The clinical trial was conducted by 11 doctors in 9 hospitals in Japan. A total of 111 neurotic patients, consisting of 20 inpatients and 91 outpatients, was admitted to the clinical trial. There were 49 females and 62 males ranging in age from 16 to 82 years, with a mean of 39.2 years.

As shown in table I, the experimental population of the study consisted of different types of neurotic patients. All patients selected for this trial exhibited certain target symptoms commonly found in neurotic states and were considered suitable for treatment with anti-anxiety drugs. These symptoms were: anxiety, tension, apprehension, mixed anxiety-depression and sleep disturbance.

The experimental design allowed flexibility in the dosage and duration of treatment. The drug was administered in the form of 10 and 25 mg capsules and the daily dose ranged from 10 to 150 mg (mainly 30–75 mg). The duration of treatment varied from 1 to 26 weeks (mainly 2–3 weeks).

In most patients, no other psychotropic medications were prescribed during the trial except for bedtime sedatives.

Table I. Patient population (age, 16–82; average 39.2 years)

	Number of patients
Inpatient	20
Outpatient	91
Sex	
Female	49
Male	62
Diagnosis	
Neurosis	
Anxiety	39
Hysterical	5
Phobic	3
Obsessive compulsive	6
Depressive	21
Depersonalization syndrome	1
Hypochondrical	24
Others (writer's cramp)	2
Personality disorder	4
Psychosomatic disorder	6
Total	111

Results and Discussion

Results, based on clinical global impressions, are summarized in table II. When therapeutic results were graded according to the overall response of the 111 patients treated, 28.8% were rated as good, 24.3% as fair, 32.4% as unchanged and 14.4% as worse. There was some improvement in 59 (53.2%) patients. Results were little influenced by inpatient-outpatient status, and no distinct differences on overall efficacy between female and male patients were found.

As shown in table III, the best results were seen in depressive neurosis. In these patients, it seemed that the primary changes related to the drug showed mainly in depressive mood, anxiety, impaired ability to concentrate and somatic complaints such as anorexia, headache and palpitation.

While about one half of patients suffering from anxiety neurosis, hypochondriacal neurosis, personality disorders and psychosomatic diseases

Table II. Results of clinical global impression

	Good		Fair	Unchanged	Worse
Inpatient	6	(11)	7	6	1
Outpatient	26	(46)	20	30	15
Female patient	17	(28)	11	15	6
Male patient	15	(31)	16	21	10
Total	32	(59)	27	36	16

Improved results are given in parentheses.

Table III. Therapeutic results in diagnostic categories

Diagnosis	Good	Fair	Unchanged	Worse
Neurosis				
Anxiety	13 (33.3)	6 (15.4)	13	7
Hysterical	1 (20.0)	1 (20.0)	2	1
Phobic		1 (33.3)	1	1
Obsessive compulsive		1 (16.7)	4	1
Depressive	8 (38.1)	9 (42.9)	3	1
Depersonalization syndrome			1	
Hypochondriacal	2 (33.3)	8 (33.3)	6	5
Others	5 (20.8)			
Personal disorder	2 (100)	1 (25.0)	2	
Psychosomatic diseases	1 (25.0)		4	

Percentages are given in parentheses.

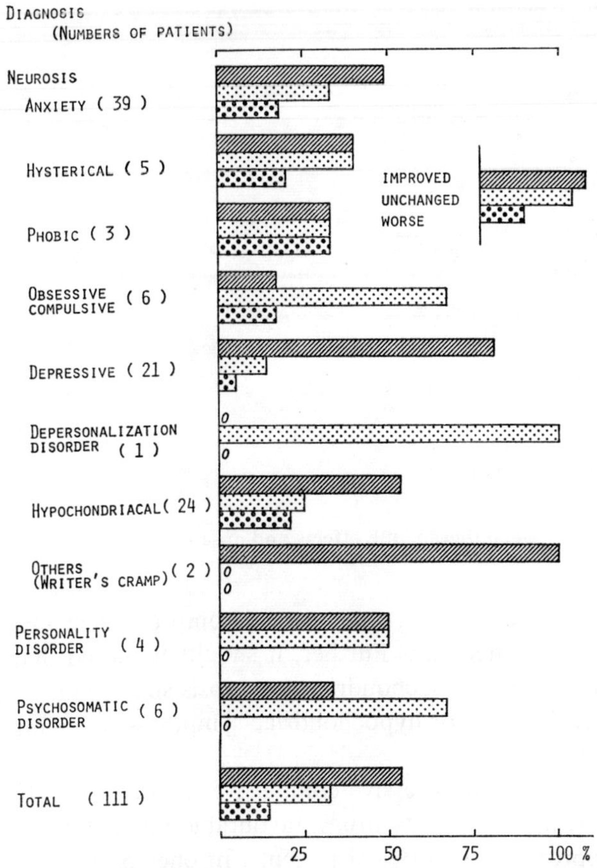

Fig. 1. Therapeutic results of trazodone.

Table IV. Therapeutic results of varying dosages

Daily dose, mg	Good	Fair	Unchanged	Worse
Less than 50	20	11	18	6
51–100	11	11	15	7
101–150	1	5	3	3

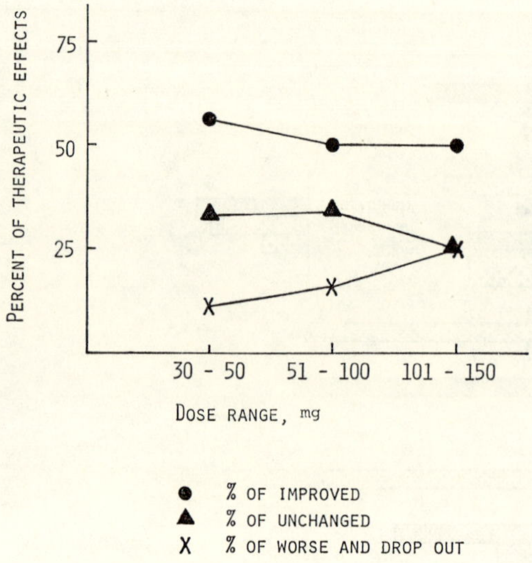

Fig. 2. Relationship between therapeutic effects and dose range.

showed favorable effects to the drug treatment, the improvement rate was especially good in anxiety neurosis. Further, it should be noted that 15–20 % of anxiety neurosis and hypochondriacal neurosis showed an exacerbation of anxiety, tension and/or hypochondriac symptoms following trazodone administration.

In hysterical neurosis and obsessive compulsive neurosis, which generally do not respond to anti-anxiety drugs, favourable therapeutic effects were obtained in approximately 40 % of patients. In one patient suffering of writer's cramp a marked reduction of finger tremor (when writing), anxiety and tension were observed. However, any conclusive remark on this findings needs to be further substantiated.

Table IV shows the therapeutic effects to varying doses of trazodone. It can be seen that changes in drug regimen did not alter improvement rates.

Adverse Effects and Laboratory Findings

Adverse reactions recorded during the trial are listed in table V. There were 12 different symptoms in 28 patients (25.2 % of the total patients). The most frequent symptoms were drowsiness, tiredness, dizziness and dry mouth. As a rule, these adverse effects were mild and transient, and none

Table V. Adverse effects

Adverse reactions	Number of patients
Drowsiness	11
Tiredness	5
Dizziness	4
Ataxia	1
Headache	1
Blurred vision	1
Increased sweating	1
Dry mouth	4
Nausea	3
Anorexia	2
Gastric pain	1
Other CI discomfort	2

of them required discontinuation of trazodone administration. This finding supports the results obtained by a number of previous workers.

Results of laboratory studies, including blood cell count, routine urinalysis and liver function, did not reveal any abnormalities in the course of trazodone treatment.

Conclusion

All the above findings suggest that trazodone has a therapeutic effect in the treatment of neurotic patients. Furthermore, an excellent tolerance when given at daily dose levels of 10–150 mg was confirmed.

The therapeutic indication of trazodone in the various neurotic disorders has not been clearly defined as yet. In the reported clinical trial, the favorable effects were most apparent in depressive neurosis and were inconsistent in other types of neurotic disorders. In order to establish the therapeutic efficacy of trazodone in anxiety neurosis, a double-blind controlled study of trazodone with diazepam and placebo is now under way.

Author's address: Dr. S. MIURA, MD, Neuropsychiatry, School of Medicine, Kitasato University, *Sagamihara* (Japan)

Free Communications Session

Chairman: D. WHEATLEY

Trazodone. Mod. Probl. Pharmacopsychiat., vol. 9, pp. 146–156,
ed. Th. A. Ban, Montreal, Que., and B. Silvestrini, Rome (Karger, Basel 1974)

Sedative and Anxiety-Reducing Properties of Trazodone

Psychophysiological Investigations with Special Reference to the Application of Pupillographic Methods

D. SCHWARZ and M. BLENDL

Max-Planck-Institut für Psychiatrie (Direktor: Prof. D. PLOOG), München

In evaluating agents with minor tranquilizing properties two factors are of special interest: (1) the extent to which they influence vigilance, and (2) their ability to reduce anxiety reactions.

Therapeutic indications depend on the relation between these two properties, which to a differing extent are combined in such substances. In many tranquilizing drugs the sedative component is relatively strong, so the use of the agent is limited.

Another important property is the time course of the sedative effects. Unfortunately, informations on the time profile often are very poor and lack an objective background. Data concerning blood levels can be transferred only with caution to the clinical effects.

These problems were investigated in a double-blind study with 20 male volunteers receiving either a placebo or 50 mg of trazodone. The study included psychological tests, electronic pupillography and polygraphic recordings of EEG, HR, respiration, photoplethysmogram and psychogalvanic skin response.

This report is based on findings obtained by the application of pupillographic methods.

The experiments were conducted using an electronic system from Polymetric Co. (fig. 1). This system contains an image transducer, a single analyzer circuit, a chart recorder and a video monitor unit. The image transducer is composed of an optical lens element and a video tube. The lens projects an image of the subject's pupil into the receiving surface on the video tube. This image is transformed into sequential electrical signals that are subsequently transformed and analyzed to yield a new signal, whose magnitude is directly proportional to the pupil diameter. The pupil's images

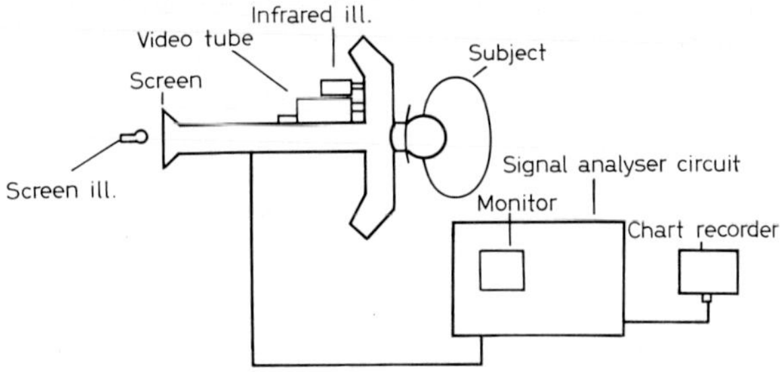

Fig. 1. Pupillometric monitoring system.

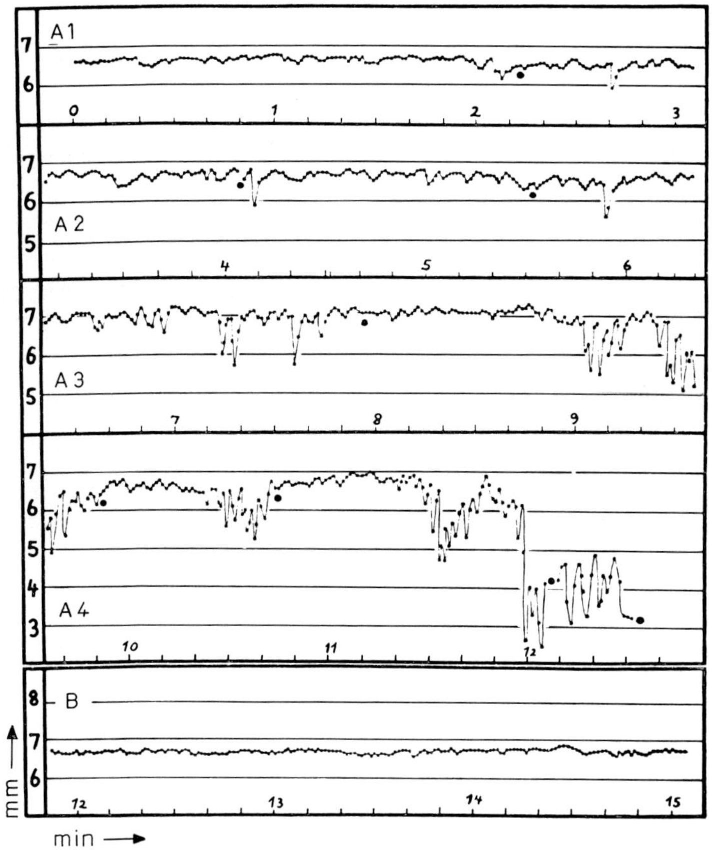

Fig. 2. Spontaneous oscillations of pupillary diameter in a person with chronic fatigue (A) and after recovery (B) [LOWENSTEIN *et al.*, 1963].

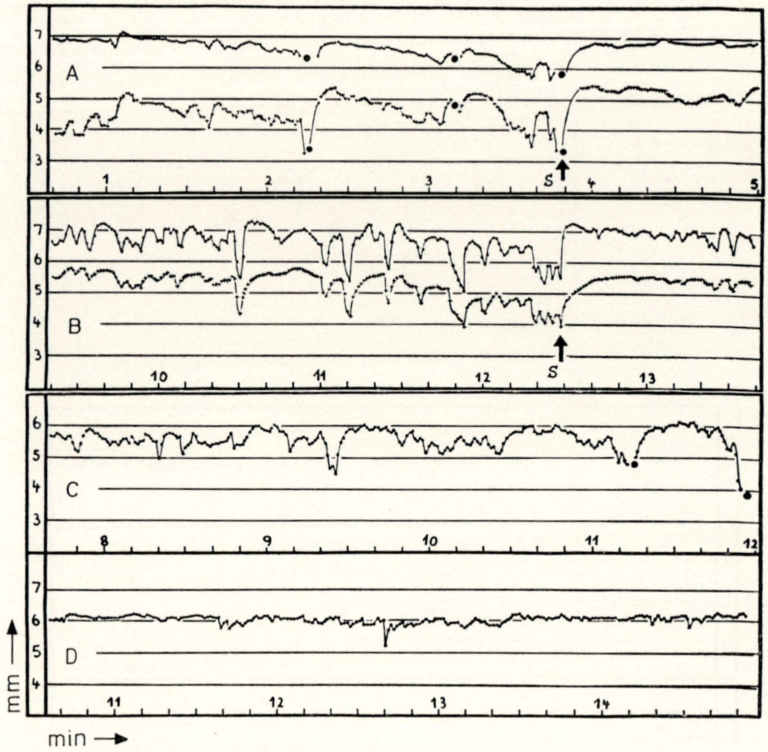

Fig. 3. Effect of amphetamine (D) on pupillary oscillation in a drowsy person (B, C) [LOWENSTEIN *et al.*, 1963].

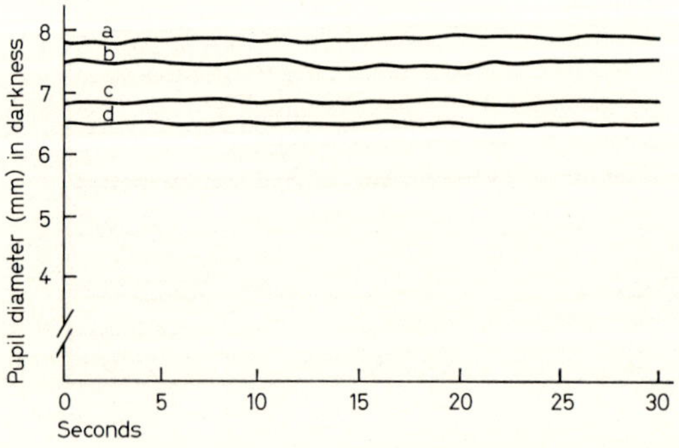

Fig. 4. Pupillary behaviour in different stages of drowsiness.

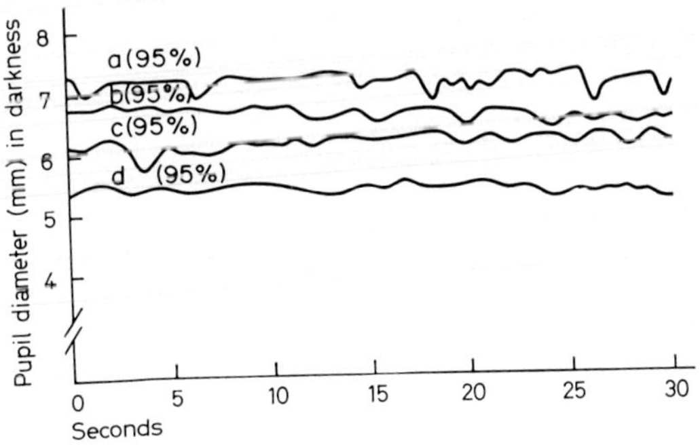

Fig. 5

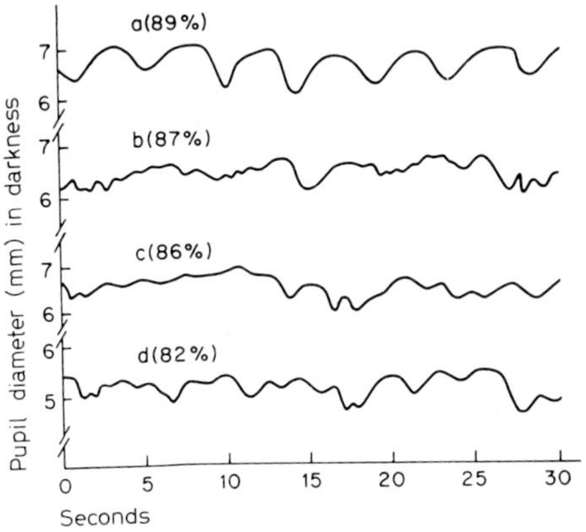

Fig. 6

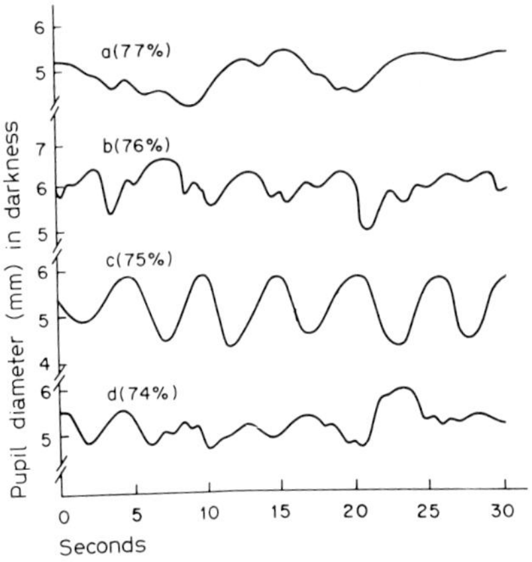

Fig. 7. From Yoss *et al.* [1970].

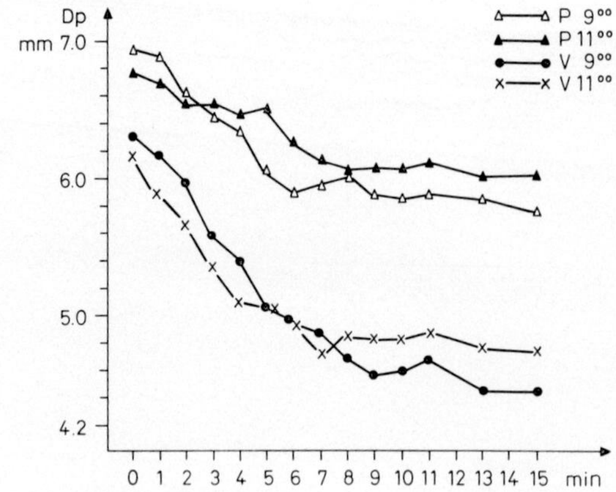

Fig. 8. Pupil diameter following application of either placebo (P) or 50 mg trazodone (V) during 15 min of reduced sensory input (n = 20).

on the video tube are scanned at a rate of 60/sec. The pupil is illuminated by infrared light, diffuse in character. By this system we obtain a continuous recording of the actual pupil size.

The aim of our first experiment was to determine the degree to which vigilance is reduced by the substance.

As LOWENSTEIN *et al.* have demonstrated in 1963, reduced wakefulness leads to a pupillary constriction and the appearance of oscillations in pupil size. As one can see in figure 2 there is a marked difference of pupillary behaviour in a person with chronic fatigue after a surgical intervention and in the same person 2 years later after complete recovery. In figure 3 LOWENSTEIN has demonstrated the effect of amphetamine on pupillary movements in an exhausted person.

YOSS *et al.* [1970] have studied such effects more systematically. They correlated clinical and behavioural information on the degree of wakefulness with pupillographic recordings and developed a classification beginning with A 'alert and sharp' unto H 'asleep, not dreaming'. The degree of reduced vigilance is defined by pupillary constriction and the amplitude of the oscillations (fig. 4–7).

In our experiment the pupil diameter was measured during 15 min in a situation of reduced sensory input. Data were obtained at about 30 and 150 min following administration of either placebo or trazodone. As one can see in figure 8 there is a marked reduction of pupil size after trazodone

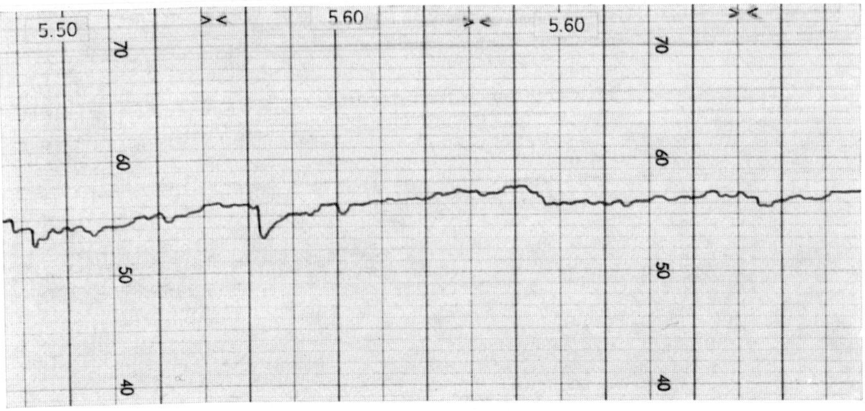

a

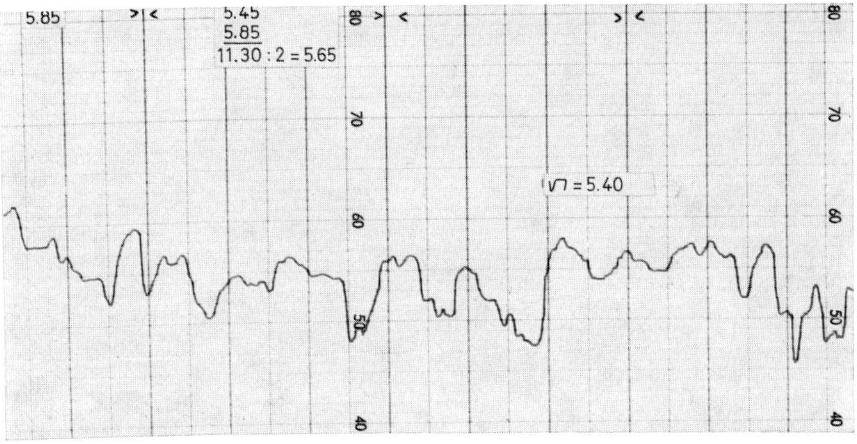

b

Fig. 9. a Pupillary behaviour 30 min after application of placebo. *b* Pupillary behaviour 30 min after application of 50 mg trazodone.

in both time samples. The reduction of pupil size during trazodone compared with placebo reaches 11–17 % in the first minute and 23–30 % after 15 min. The differences are highly significant. At the same time slow waves of high amplitude appear (fig. 9).

Following Yoss *et al.* [1970] the observed changes correspond to a relatively slight reduction of vigilance according to the pupillographic stages C and D. This result is also confirmed by ratings of subjective wakefulness demonstrating a significant sedative effect 45, 90, 135 and 180 min after trazodone administration (fig. 10).

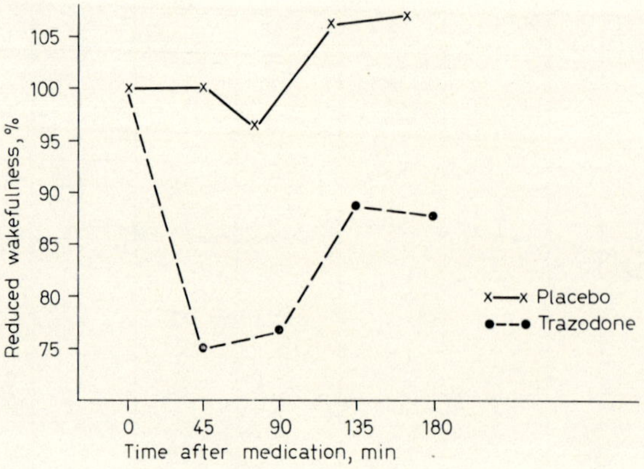

Fig. 10. Rating of reduced subjective wakefulness following placebo or trazodone (n = 20).

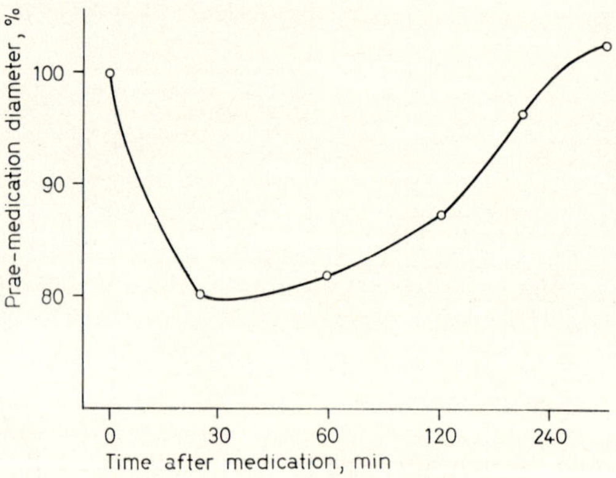

Fig. 11. Pupil diameter following application of 50 mg trazodone (n = 5).

As the first study showed there was a very early onset of the effect and no significant change during 3 h. We were, therefore, interested in obtaining a more objective and precise time profile of sedative effects in a second experiment. In 5 subjects pupillographic recordings were obtained by frequent measurements. The rapid onset of sedative effect was confirmed: it is remarkable between 20 and 30 min following administration with only slight variability between individuals (fig. 11). Between the first and third hour there is a maximum effect with only poor variance. Three hours after

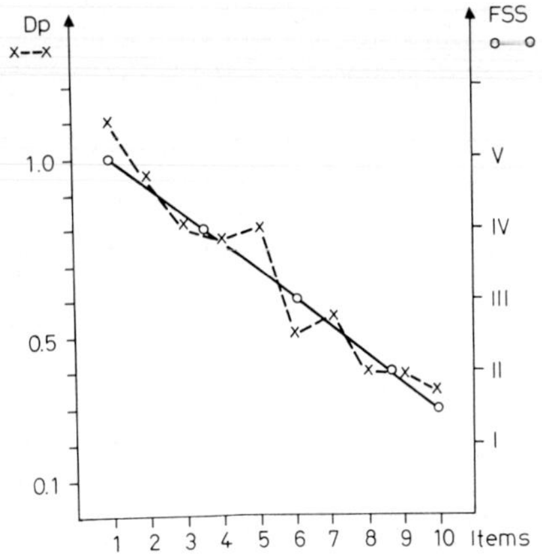

Fig. 12. Comparison of pupillary reflex dilation (Dp) on anxiety-producing items and ratings of anxiety on the fear survey schedule (FSS) by WOLPE.

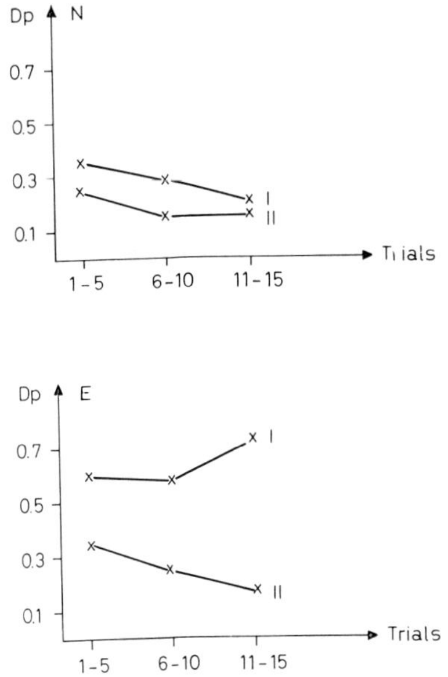

Fig. 13. Pupillary reflex dilation on neutral (N) and emotional (E) items before (I) and after (II) behaviour modification of phobic patients (n = 4).

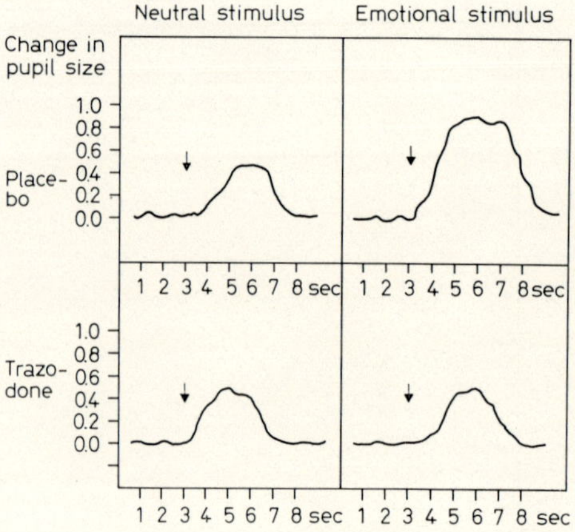

Fig. 14. Pupillary reflex dilation on neutral and emotional items in one subject after application of placebo and trazodone.

Table I. Pupillary dilation (mm) during neutral (N) and emotional (E) stimulation (n = 16)

	E	N	
V	0.5	0.5	n. s.
P	0.9	0.6	$p < 0.02$
	$p < 0.01$	n. s.	

trazodone administration the effect slowly diminishes and goes to zero at about 4–5 h later.

The third experiment was performed to obtain information on the anxiety reducing properties of the agent. According to HESS [1972] and others pupillographic recordings have proved to be a very sensitive instrument for evaluating emotional reactiveness. In contrast to the light reflex of the pupil the so-called psychosensory reflex leads to a dilation following an emotional stimulus with a latency of about 0.3 sec.

As JANISSE [1973] pointed out: (1) pupil reaction is always one of dilation to an emotional stimulus, and (2) pupil size is related to the intensity of an emotion.

In previous studies we demonstrated that there is a strong correlation between pupillary dilatation and times rated as 'high' or 'low' anxiety provoking in the FSS by Wolpe (fig. 12). The dilation following emotional stimuli, compared with neutral items, was reduced after behaviour therapy of phobics (fig. 13).

To evaluate the anxiety-reducing properties of trazodone, subjects were asked to imagine three items they had previously rated as high anxiety provoking and three items they considered neutral in the FSS.

In figure 14 pupillary reactions of one subject during the conditions neutral-placebo, neutral-trazodone, emotional-placebo, emotional-trazodone are demonstrated. As one can see, in all cases there is a slight dilation of the pupil, caused by the imagery task. But the reaction on the emotional item during placebo is much more pronounced. During trazodone there is no difference in the reaction to emotional items compared with neutral items. This means that the anxiety provoking effect of those items have vanished following the application of trazodone.

The averaged reactions of all subjects are shown in table I. After trazodone there is a nearly complete and significant reduction of emotional reactions to items formerly rated as anxiety provoking. In summary: Continuous polygraphic recordings were performed during 45–120 min after trazodone administration. In accordance with the only slight sedative effects observed in the pupillogram there were no gross changes in the EEG. There was also no difference in HR comparing placebo and trazodone, neither in a relaxing situation nor during noise stimulation. Respiratory rate and peripheral circulation remained unchanged. A self-rating concerning 18 different bodily sensations did not show any important side-effects, with the exception of slight weakness.

Our investigations lead to the following conclusions: (1) in a dosage of 50 mg *per os* trazodone has no relevant side-effects – there were no changes in heart rate, peripheral circulation, respiration and EEG; (2) trazodone has significant, but only slight effects on vigilance; (3) the onset of sedative effects is quite rapid, beginning 20–30 min after medication and lasts for 4–5 h, and (4) trazodone has marked anxiety-reducing effects.

In preliminary investigations on psychiatric patients the experimental results could be confirmed. Trazodone proved to be a tranquilizing agent with minimal side-effects and only slight influence on vigilance, at the same time exerting excellent effects on affective hyper-reactiveness.

References

HESS, E. T.: Pupillometrics. A method of studying mental emotional and sensory processes; in GREENFIELD and STERNBACH Handbook of psychophysiology (Holt, Rinehart & Winston, London 1972).

JANISSE, M. T.: Pupil size and effect. Proc. Coll. on the Pupil, 1973.

LOWENSTEIN, O., *et al.:* Pupillary movements during acute and chronic fatigue. Invest. Ophthal. *2:* 138–157 (1963).

SCHWARZ, D.: Problems in identifying emotional stimuli by pupillographic recordings. Proc. 8th Coll. on the Pupil, 1973.

YOSS, R., *et al.:* Pupil size and spontaneous pupillary waves associated with alertness, drowsiness and sleep. Neurology *20:* 545–554 (1970).

Author's address: Dr. D. SCHWARZ, Max-Planck-Institut für Psychiatrie, *D-8000 München* (FRG)

Trazodone. Mod. Probl. Pharmacopsychiat., vol. 9, pp. 157–159,
ed. Th. A. Ban, Montreal, Que., and B. Silvestrini, Rome (Karger, Basel 1974)

Clinical Experience with Trazodone in the Treatment of Psychiatric Patients

A. LOPEZ ZANON

Director, Hospital F. Franco, Madrid

Trazodone is the first s. triazolo-(4,3-a)-pyridine derivative which has passed the screening for use in therapeutic psychiatry [3]. This product was supplied to us under the trade name Hubberdone for clinical experimentation. We received 25, 50 and 100 mg capsules for use in hospitalized patients and for outpatients. From a pharmacological point of view, trazodone showed antiserotonin activity without producing extrapyramidal manifestations [5].

After reading an excellent report [6] we followed a therapeutic regimen using progressively increasing doses, up to 600 mg/patient/day. Our case series consisted of 20 patients ranging in age from 11 to 71 years. No undesirable side-effects were observed in any of the patients. In the cases where we used a precursor of serotonin, under double-blind conditions, we administered it orally in a dose averaging between 50 and 100 mg/patient/day. The therapeutic effects were evaluated by means of the Hamilton Depression Rating Scale (HAM) and the Brief Psychiatric Rating Scale of Overall and Gorham (BPRS).

The cases studied in this trial can be summarized as follows:

Schizophrenic psychosis (8 cases). Case 1, male, 28 years old, residual schizophrenia, fair improvement; case 2, male, 50 years old, chronic paranoid psychosis, no improvement; case 3, male, 27 years old, incipient schizophrenia, excellent results; case 4, male, 25 years old, schizophrenia, no improvement; case 5, male, 33 years old, paranoid psychosis, fair improvement; case 6, female, 29 years old, schizophrenia, fair improvement; case 7, female, 32 years old, residual schizophrenia, no improvement; and case 8, female, 40 years old, paranoid psychosis, fair improvement.

Hypochondriac syndromes (2 cases). Case 1, male, 44 years old, hypochondriacal neurosis with symptoms of paranoia, excellent results; and case 2, female, 42 years old, depressive hypochondriasis, no improvement.

Involutional depression (4 cases). Case 1, male, 58 years old, involutional depression, excellent results; case 2, female, 71 years old, involutional depression, excellent results; case 3, male, 68 years old, involutional depression, excellent results, and case 4, female, 61 years old, involutional depression, excellent results.

Organic psychosis (1 case). Case 1, male, 67 years old, Pick's disease, marked improvement.

Psychosomatic disorders (1 case). Case 1, female, 66 years old, astasia-abasia, excellent results.

Reactive depressions (2 cases). Case 1, male, 56 years old, reactive depression, no improvement, and case 2, female, 32 years old, endoreactive depression, marked improvement.

Other psychoses (2 cases). Case 1, male, 11 years old, obsessive-compulsive psychosis, excellent results, and case 2, female, 14 years old, anorexia nervosa, fair improvement.

As can be seen, the product was effective in involutional depressions, in which, according to the data obtained, it exerted its effect by its anti-serotonin activity. In schizophrenia, the results cannot be considered favorable. However, perhaps it is necessary to carry out further investigation for longer periods of time.

Rather remarkable results were obtained in the case of Pick's disease, naturally referring to the improvement of the patient's behavior.

Our experience is still limited, but nevertheless we think that trazodone has a well deserved place among the psychotropic agents, especially in hypochondriacal neurosis, obsessive-compulsive neurosis, involutional depression, psychosomatic disorders.

Before concluding we like to draw attention to a fact that is of great interest. Our previous experience [2] demonstrated the efficacy of a precursor of serotonin (α-ketoglutarate of L-5-hydroxytryptophane) in the treatment of involutional depression. It was a coincidence to demonstrate that the clinical action of trazodone can be correlated with its antiserotonin activity. We had four patients under treatment with the above-mentioned precursor of serotonin and after already obtaining a moderate improvement we began to use trazodone in two of the patients. As a result all signs of improvement suddenly disappeared. This unexpected event prompted us to begin a double-blind trial on all the four patients affected with involutional depression. We could thus demonstrate that both products (the precursor of serotonin and trazodone) were effective when employed separately. The employment of both drugs together was followed by an increase in the severity of the symptoms to the point where one can state that both drugs were ineffective when used together. Perhaps it would, therefore, be very interesting to carry out a trial with probenecid [4] before deciding which drug is to be used in a depressed patient.

References

1 FREYHAN, F. A.: Neuro-psychopharmacology, vol. 2 (Elsevier, Amsterdam 1961).

2 LOPEZ ZANON, A.: Comunicación preliminar sobre el empleo de una nueva sal del 5-hydroxitriptofano en psiquiatría. Cuad. Madrileños Psiquiat. *4:* 25–38 (1973).

3 PALAZZO, G.: Chemistry of Trazodone. Round Table Discussion: Trazodone, a New Psychotropic Agent, Amsterdam 1973. Curr. Ther. Res. *15:* 745–748 (1973).

4 PRAAG, H. M. VAN and KORF, J.: Aspects of depression. Proc. Symp. World Psychiatric Ass., Madrid 1972, pp. 149–156 (Sadac, Barcelona 1973).

5 SILVESTRINI, B. and LISCIANI, R.: Pharmacology of Trazodone. Round Table Discussion: Trazodone, a New Psychotropic Agent, Amsterdam 1973. Curr. Ther. Res. *15:* 749–754 (1973).

6 UCHA UDABE, R.: Clinical experience with a new psychotropic drug, Trazodone: a review of literature. Round Table Discussion: Trazodone, a New Psychotropic Agent, Amsterdam 1973. Curr. Ther. Res. *15:* 755–763 (1973).

Author's address: Dr. A. LOPEZ ZANON, Cea Bermudez 10, *Madrid* (Spain)

Trazodone. Med. Probl. Pharmacopsychiat., vol. 9, pp. 160–166,
ed. Th. A. Ban, Montreal, Que., and B. Silvestrini, Rome (Karger, Basel 1974)

EEG Findings in Geriatric Patients Treated with Trazodone

R. MONTANINI

Ospedale Civile F. Ghiringhelli, Gallarate, Varese

Electroencephalography is one of the methods currently used for a better assessment of psychotropic drugs both at the experimental and at the clinical level.

A periodical EEG control during the course of therapy gives valuable information about the tolerance, mechanism of action and possibly the site of action of drugs.

It is for these reasons that we considered it important to carry out an electroencephalographic study of trazodone in man. The following procedures were used: (a) acute intravenous administration of the drug in adults with neurotic depression; (b) repeated EEG recordings during oral therapy in adults with neurotic depression; (c) repeated EEG recordings during oral drug therapy in geriatric patients (over 65 years of age).

Results

Group A. This group was comprised of adults with neurotic depression without organic changes.

A continuous EEG recording was made before, during and for a period of 4 h after slow intravenous administration (carried out over 5 min) of 1 mg/kg of trazodone. Heart rate and blood pressure were also controlled periodically. In all patients, immediately following the i. v. injection there was a decrease in both systolic and diastolic blood pressures lasting for 10–15 min. The drop was 20–30 mm Hg for the systolic pressure and slightly less for the diastolic.

The following readings were obtained: in 50% of the patients ex-

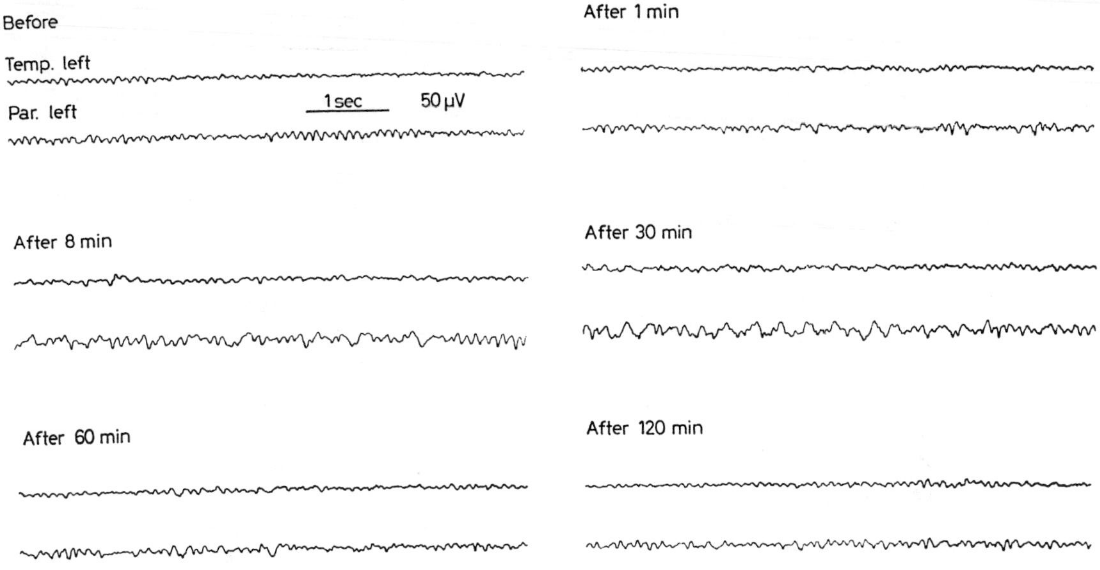

Fig. 1. Immediate recordings during 120 min following trazodone administration (50 mg i. v.).

amined no important changes were observed; only continuous, regular low voltage waves with high frequency (15–18 c/s) were seen in the prefrontal regions. There was also a slight decrease in α-wave activity.

In the other 50% of patients, 7–8 min after the injection of the drug, high voltage slow waves were observed at a frequency of 4–5 c/s with the persistence, however, of α-activity. After 30 min the slow waves became continuous (fig. 1). The EEG changes due to trazodone disappeared 2–3 h after the injection.

Group B. 43 patients ranging in age from 20 to 65 were admitted to this group. They presented mainly with neurotic depression, without any important organic lesions of the nervous system.

These patients were treated with oral trazodone in doses ranging from 75 to 200 mg per day. EEG controls were carried out after 8, 15 and 30 days of treatment.

The EEG tracings before treatment were normal since patients showing important EEG abnormalities were excluded from this group.

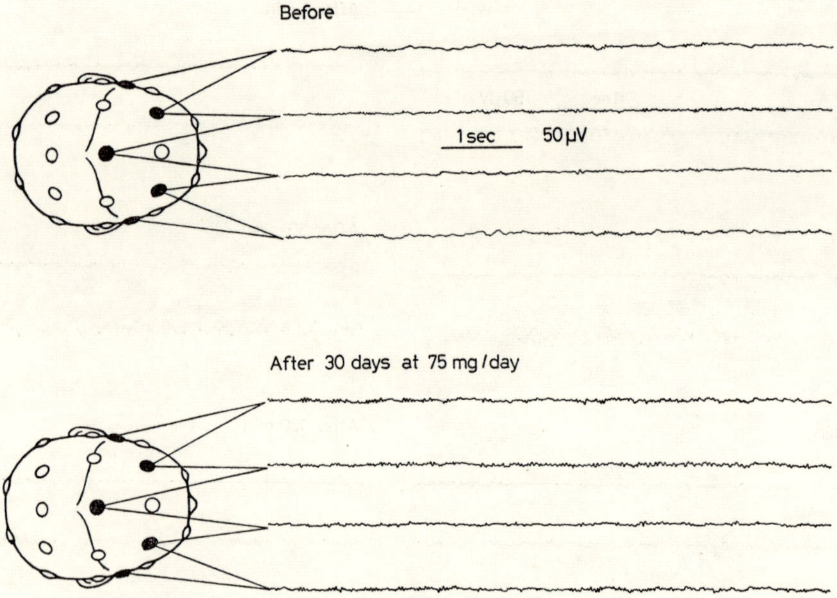

Fig. 2. Recordings from a 50-year-old patient before and 30 days after administration of trazodone.

During treatment with trazodone no conspicuous variations were observed. In about one third of the cases the appearance of almost continuous, fast, low voltage waves in the prefrontal areas was noted (fig. 2).

Only in 10 % of the cases was the basal frequency activity slightly lower. Slow activity theta or delta waves never appeared.

Group C. This group consisted of 25 patients over 65 years of age with neurological and psychiatric conditions attributable to diffuse cerebral arteriosclerosis: mild neurological disturbances, memory deficit, difficulty in concentration, insufficient emotional control, anxiety, disturbances of the wakefulness and sleep pattern, slight confusional states, slight depression.

These symptoms were mainly caused by cerebral arteriosclerosis, although they could have been partly attributed to environmental situations.

Fig. 3. EEG recordings in a 75-year-old patient before and after treatment with trazodone (75 mg/day p. o.).

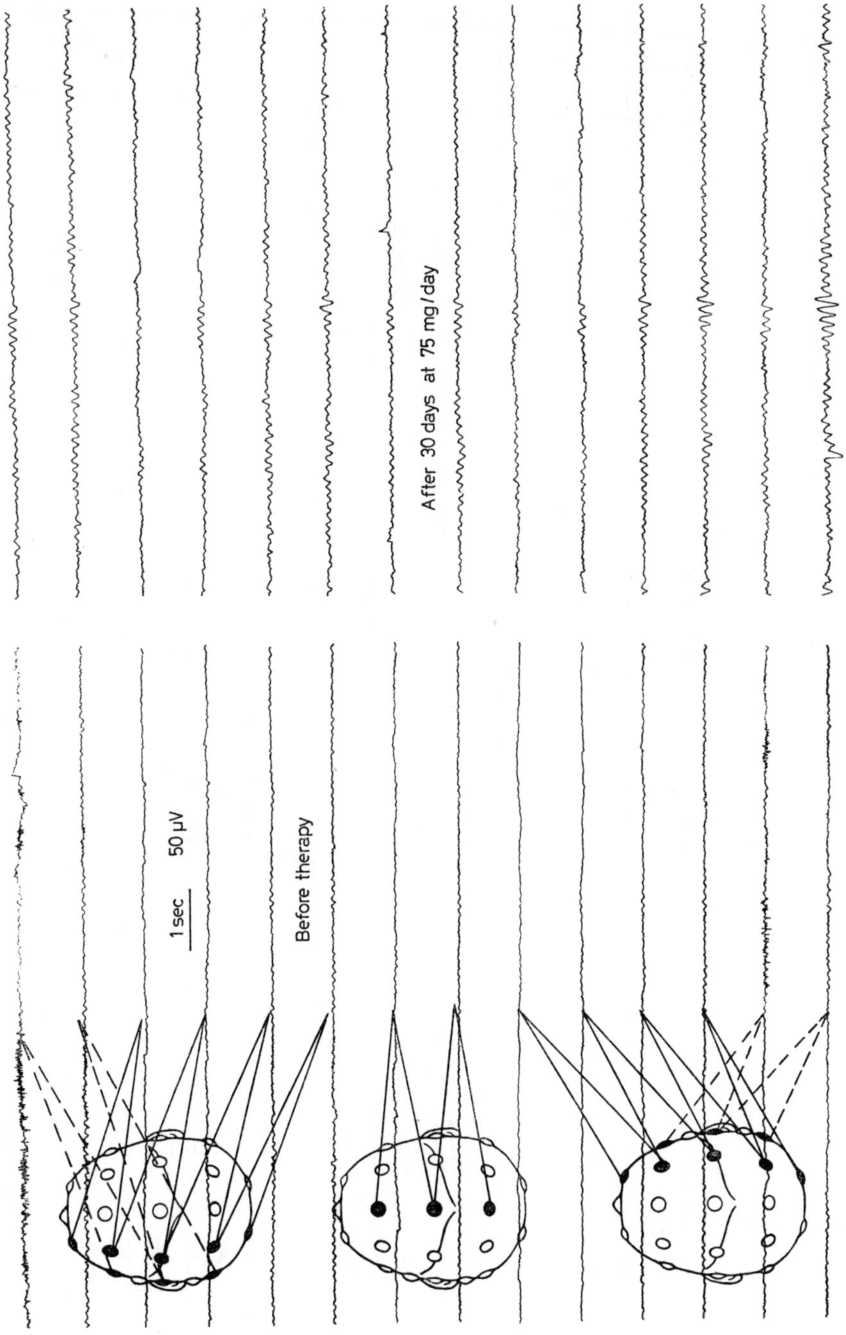
1 sec
50 µV
Before therapy
After 30 days at 75 mg/day

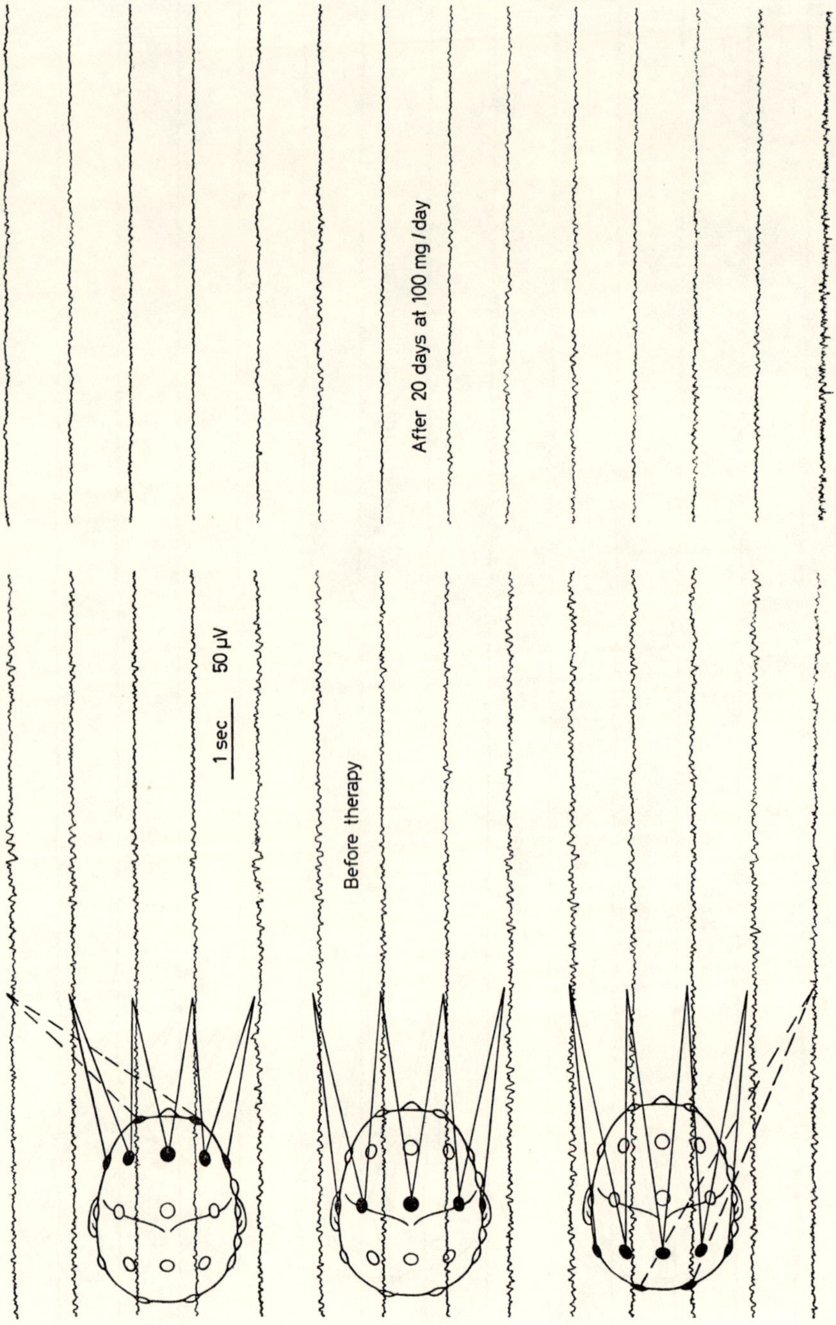

After 20 days at 100 mg / day
1 sec
50 µV
Before therapy

All patients examined were recovered in a nursing home.

Patients with marked biochemical abnormalities or severe clinical changes were excluded.

Treatment consisted of 75 mg of trazodone p. o. per day. EEG recordings were taken prior to commencement of therapy and after 30 days of treatment.

The basal EEG was considered to be normal only in 6 cases. In the other patients there were abnormalities which are often found in cerebral arteriosclerosis and in old age: low frequency, low voltage alpha rhythm and even flat recordings, were observed as well as irregular theta waves.

20 % of the recordings showed no variations during treatment with trazodone. In 45 % of the cases, fast low voltage activity was observed in the prefrontal region. This finding was quite obvious in half of these cases (equal to 20 % of the total number of patients in this study) and hardly noticeable in the other half. In 33 % of the cases, an increase in the voltage of the basal rhythm was observed. In 20 % of all patients the alpha rhythm, which was of very low voltage and low frequency, became more rapid and regular. Occasionally the frequency diminished slightly.

In 10 % of the patients a slight but appreciable decrease of the slow activity, present before treatment, was noted. Considering the overall picture of the EEG findings, there was an improvement of the recordings in about one quarter of those examined. This improvement is represented by a decrease of the slow pathological activity and by an increase of the α-activity.

In 25 % of all cases the frequency of the α-rhythm showed a tendency to slowing down markedly, whereas in none of the patients pathological type of activity was ever noted, i. e. delta or theta waves appeared (unless present prior to commencement of therapy).

Discussion

EEG findings demonstrate that: (a) the activity of trazodone can be proven by electrophysiological techniques; (b) the most common changes in the EEG are characterized by an increased activity in the prefrontal areas

---

Fig. 4. EEG recordings before and after therapy in a 70-year-old patient treated with trazodone (100 mg/day p. o.).

as seen with the benzodiazepines, the barbiturates, meprobamate and amitryptiline; (c) improvements in EEG tracings of geriatric patients suffering from cerebral arteriosclerosis was obtained in 25 % of cases.

Trazodone produced an improvement of the EEG tracing not only by synchronizing the rhythm but also by increasing the frequency of the α-waves and decreasing the number of pathological waves. EEG changes were neither age related nor attributable to a variation in the psychic state of the patients. In other words, improvement on the alpha rhythm cannot be ascribed only to a decrease of the anxiety factor.

Other drugs which cause even greater sedation do not usually produce the above mentioned EEG changes especially in patients with cerebral arteriosclerosis. Trazodone generally produced greater changes or improvements of the EEG in geriatric patients than did other psychotropic agents.

References

BAN, T. A.; LEHMANN, H. E.; AMIN, M.; GALVAN, L.; NAIR, N. P.; VERGARA, L., and ZOCH, C.: Comprehensive clinical studies with trazodone. Curr. ther. Res. *15:* 540–551 (1973).

BOVET, D.; LONGO, V. G. et SILVESTRINI, B.: Les méthodes d'investigations électrophysiologiques dans l'étude des médicaments tranquillisants; in Psychotropic drugs, p. 139 (Elsevier, London 1957).

CAZZULLO, C. L.: Communication at the Conference on EEG and human Psychopharmacology. World Congr. Psychiatry (Max Fink, Montreal 1961).

MONTANINI, R. and RAVASINI, C.: Psychopharmacologic treatment in relation with electroencephalography. Med. Exp. *5:* 396–405 (1961).

MONTANINI, R. e RAVASINI, C.: Contributo dell'elettroencefalografia allo studio delle associazioni fra farmaci psicotropi. Riv. Neurol. *34:* 359–367 (1964).

MONTANINI, R.: Metabolismo e interazione fra farmaci. Quaderni di Neuropsicofarmacologia (Ed. Soc. Ital. Neuropsicofarmacologia, Milano 1971).

SILVESTRINI, B.; CIOLI, V.; BURBERI, S., and CATANESE, B.: Pharmacological properties of AF 1161 a new psychotropic drug. Int. J. Neuropharmacol. *7:* 587–599 (1968).

Author's address: Prof. R. MONTANINI, Ospedale Civile S. Antonio Abate, *Gallarate, Varese* (Italy)

Trazodone. Mod. Probl. Pharmacopsychiat., vol. 9, pp. 167–172,
ed. Th. A. Ban, Montreal, Que., and B. Silvestrini, Rome (Karger, Basel 1974)

Trazodone's Effects on Patients with Partial or Total Ventilatory Insufficiency

G. Gunella

Servizio di Fisiopatologia Respiratoria e Terapia Medica dell'Insufficienza Respiratoria, Policlinico S. Orsola, Bologna

Whoever deals with respiratory physiopathology knows very well that in patients with chronic respiratory insufficiency the appearance of a series of symptoms such as psychomotor agitation, time and space disorientation, irritability and nocturnal insomnia are indicative in general of an early stage of respiratory encephalopathy. The presence of arterial hypoxemia and hypercapnia in these patients confirms the diagnosis.

Unfortunately, these symptoms aren't often interpreted as an early stage of respiratory encephalopathy; generally these symptoms are considered as the expression of 'nervous breakdown'.

This incorrect diagnosis results in a wrong therapy, i. e. the administration of barbiturates or tranquilizers. This in turn causes a considerable aggravation of the respiratory state of the patient with a consequent onset of a comatous state.

It is important in this connection to point out that patients with chronic respiratory insufficiency (such as chronic bronchitic, emphysematous and asthmatic patients in the phase of chronic hypercapnia) already show a depression of respiratory centers owing to the existing hypercapnia. It is therefore sufficient to administer to these patients low doses of barbiturates or tranquilizers to deteriorate the depression of the respiratory centers thus giving rise to a respiratory coma.

Figure 1 shows what can happen to an emphysematous patient who received 1 g of meprobamate at home.

On admission to the ward, the patient was precomatous with a $PaCO_2$ of 75 mm Hg, an arterial pH of 7.25 and a total plasmatic CO_2 content of 77 % in volume (case one).

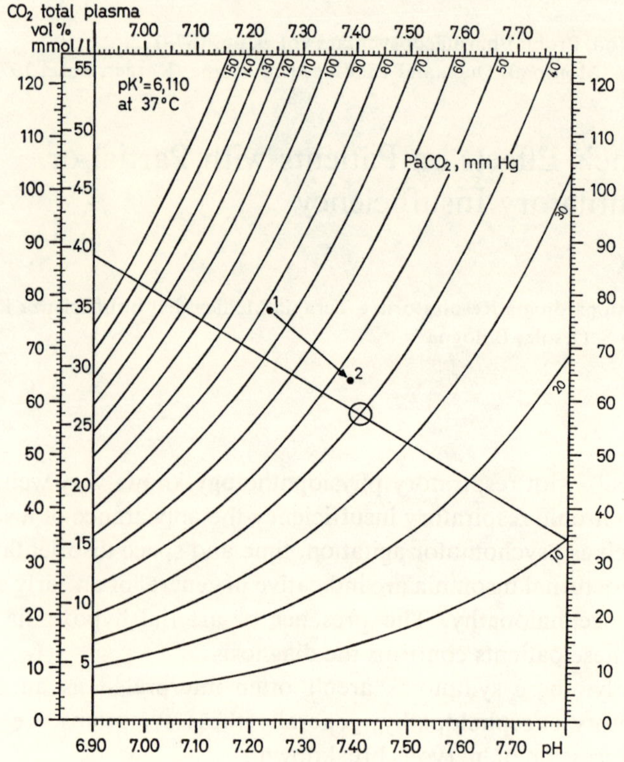

Fig. 1. Respiratory depression after 1 g of meprobamate in a patient with pulmonary emphysema. Point 1 on the Davenport's diagram shows the hemogasanalytical situation after 1 g of meprobamate; point 2 shows the improvement of the respiratory insufficiency after 72 h of artificial ventilation.

This severe ventilatory depression was corrected by means of artificial ventilation: $PaCO_2$ was lowered to 47 mm Hg; arterial pH increased to 7.38 and total plasmatic CO_2 reached 63 % in volume.

This example illustrates the considerable risk of aggravation involved in the administration of tranquilizers even at low dosages to patients with respiratory insufficiency: the same can be said for barbiturates.

However, in the field of pneumology, sedatives can be useful in certain cases: for example, in asthmatic patients with considerable anxiety state and a sensation of dyspnea without hypercapnia, or hypoxemia, or disturbances of the intra-alveolar air distribution. The 'psychic' tachypnea present

Table I. Chronic emphysematous, bronchitic patients with isolated arterial hypoxemia

Case No.	Before treatment			After 6 days of treatment		
	PaO_2, mm Hg	$PaCO_2$, mm Hg	pH, u	PaO_2, mm Hg	$PaCO_2$, mm Hg	pH, u
1	68	38	7.30	72	40	7.38
2	79	40	7.38	84	41	7.38
3	86	36	7.40	85	40	7.39
4	81	41	7.41	78	41	7.40
5	75	41	7.38	81	39	7.41
6	68	38	7.37	75	39	7.38
7	89	42	7.37	90	41	7.38
8	69	38	7.41	77	40	7.38
9	62	41	7.36	66	40	7.35
10	80	37	7.38	81	38	7.40
11	80	39	7.40	79.5	39.6	7.38
12	65	36	7.37	78	36	7.38
13	56	32	7.43	58	30	7.43
14	63	31	7.40	68	34	7.39
15	76	40	7.38	78	41	7.40
16	75	37	7.38	78	40	7.40
17	71	39	7.37	70	39	7.40
18	64	37	7.38	68	38	7.38
19	78	40	7.37	86	38	7.40
20	65	40	7.37	68	42	7.38
Mean	72.1	38.3	7.38	76.2	38.8	7.38

in these patients is one of the causes of their ventilatory insufficiency; the other cause is the increase of airways resistance. In these conditions the use of low doses of tranquilizers is justified and useful; these drugs can be employed only after a careful examination of the respiratory function. It is evident that the general practitioner hardly possesses the means for performing a complete functional respiratory exploration. It is therefore necessary to have drugs which are devoid of a depressive action on the respiratory centers. With this idea in mind we wanted to investigate the possible depressing action of trazodone on the respiratory centers. We performed several investigations.

A. 20 patients (chronic bronchitic, asthmatic and emphysematous patients) suffering from ventilatory insufficiency with resting arterial hypoxemia (without hypercapnia) received a dose of 50 mg per day of trazodone for a period of 6 days.

B. Eight patients (chronic bronchitic, asthmatic and emphysematous patients) suffering from ventilatory insufficiency with resting hypoxemia and arterial hypercapnia received 50 mg per day of trazodone for a period of 3 days; in the second group of patients aminophylline was administered concomitantly with trazodone.

In all the cases, before and after the treatment, we measured: partial tension of arterial O_2 (PaO_2); partial tension of arterial CO_2 ($PaCO_2$), and arterial pH.

It is known that these functional indexes reflect the ventilatory capacity of a subject at the alveolar level.

Table I reports the arterial hemogasanalytic data of 20 patients affected by chronic ventilatory insufficiency with resting arterial hypoxemia not accompanied by hypercapnia and treated with 50 mg per day of trazodone for 6 days.

The above data clearly demonstrate that 50 mg of trazodone administered over a period of 6 days does not depress ventilation in subjects affected by chronic ventilatory insufficiency with arterial hypoxemia not accompanied by hypercapnia. In fact, even if we limit ourselves to considering the mean values of the arterial hemogasanalytic indexes the following was observed in the 20 cases: before treatment – $PaO_2 = 72.1$ mm Hg, $PaCO_2 = 38.3$ mm Hg and pH = 7.38; after 6 days of treatment with trazodone – $PaO_2 = 76.2$ mm Hg, $PaCO_2 = 38.8$ mm Hg and pH = 7.38.

Table II reports the arterial hemogasanalytic data of 8 patients affected by chronic ventilatory insufficiency with resting arterial hypoxemia and hypercapnia and treated with 50 mg per day of trazodone for 3 days concomitant with aminophylline.

Data reported in table II show that trazodone does not possess any adverse effect on ventilation: in fact, in the group of 8 patients affected by global respiratory insufficiency, i. e. with hypoxemia and arterial hypercapnia, the analysis of the mean values demonstrated: before treatment – $PaO_2 = 55.6$ mm Hg, $PaCO_2 = 50.4$ mm Hg and pH = 7.34; after treatment – $PaO_2 = 56.5$ mm Hg, $PaCO_2 = 50.1$ mm Hg and pH = 7.35.

One could object that in these 8 patients trazodone was administered only for 3 days instead of 6, as was the case in the 20 patients described in table I, and that aminophylline was this time associated with trazodone. In

Table II. Chronic bronchitic and emphysematous patients in phase of hypoxemia and arterial hypercapnia

Case No.	Before treatment			After 3 days of treatment		
	PaO_2, mm Hg	$PaCO_2$, mm Hg	pH, u	PaO_2, mm Hg	$PaCO_2$, mm Hg	pH, u
21	48	46	7.33	49	56	7.34
22	45	59	7.29	58	51	7.35
23	52	48	7.37	47	45	7.36
24	64	47	7.38	56	50	7.34
25	66	50	7.36	53	49	7.37
26	61	52	7.35	66	48	7.37
27	55.6	50.4	7.34	64	51	7.36
28	55	52	7.33	60	51	7.35
Mean	55	50	7.34	56.5	50.1	7.35

The arterial hemogasanalytical data concerning 8 patients affected by ventilatory insufficiency with resting hypoxemia and arterial hypercapnia treated for 3 days with 50 mg per day of trazodone concomitant with aminophylline are reported above.

fact, aminophylline could have eliminated the possible depressing action of trazodone on the respiratory centers. It is possible to reply to those objections by saying that if trazodone had actually depressed the respiratory centers in these 8 patients, this depression would not have been prevented by the low doses of aminophylline used: in fact, the 400 mg per day of aminophylline associated with trazodone do not have such a strong analeptic effect so as to prevent a possible depressing action of trazodone on the respiratory centers.

The test on these 8 patients was conducted for only 3 days for precautionary purposes. In fact a patient presenting with hypoxemia and hypercapnia urgently required artificial ventilation treatment. It was therefore not advisable to wait for a long time before instituting this type of treatment.

It must be added that our investigation on trazodone was not limited to what is shown in table I and II.

In fact, 9 of the 20 patients described in table I continued to receive treatment with trazodone at the dose of 50 mg per day associated with aminophylline at the dose of 800 mg per day. This treatment was continued for a period ranging from 4 to 14 days according to the condition of the patients.

Out of these 9 patients 7 improved whereas in 2 cases PaO_2, $PaCO_2$ and arterial pH were not modified. The improvement of the arterial hemogas-analytic data is naturally connected to the action of the high doses of aminophylline employed. It is this improvement that leads us to conclude that even for long-term treatments, trazodone does not exert depressing effects on the respiratory centers. Had trazodone exerted a depressing action, the high doses of aminophylline would have maintained unchanged the initial situation.

On the basis of our investigation we can state that trazodone, at a dose of 50 mg per day, does not depress the respiratory centers in patients affected by chronic ventilatory insufficiency with isolated arterial hypox-emia or accompanied by arterial hypercapnia.

It is true that in patients with hypoxemia and hypercapnia we combined aminophylline with trazodone administration; however, the doses employed were low and ultimately devoid of analeptic effect on the respiratory centers in patients presenting with hypercapnia.

It is possible that doses of trazodone higher than 50 mg per day could exert a depressing action on the respiratory centers in hypercapnic patients. We have no experience in this connection.

It is advisable to carry out a complete examination of the respiratory function whenever doses of trazodone higher than 50 mg per day are admin-istered. It is obvious that if a patient with respiratory insufficiency also presents a psychic condition, which is the manifestation of respiratory encephalopathy, treatment should not be based on the use of tranquilizers; the treatment will have to be carried out with means apt to improve the ventilatory insufficiency.

Author's address: Prof. G. GUNELLA, Servizio di Fisiopatologia Respiratoria e Terapia Medica dell'Insufficienza Respiratoria, Policlinico S. Orsola, *Bologna* (Italy)

Trazodone. Mod. Probl. Pharmacopsychiat., vol. 9, pp. 173–175,
ed. Th. A. Ban, Montreal, Que., and B. Silvestrini, Rome (Karger, Basel 1974)

Clinical Experiences with Trazodone on Various Psychoneuroses in Japan

Y. Shibahara

Psychiatric Section, Kyoto First Red Cross Hospital, Kyoto

Since 1968, we have studied the clinical effects of trazodone in patients suffering from schizophrenia, depression and neurosis. We found trazodone to be clinically effective in the control of emotional instability. The most remarkable clinically significant characteristics of trazodone lie just between those of diazepam and amitriptyline.

62 patients ranging from 20 to 68 years in age were included in this study. The patients consisted of schizophrenics admitted to a mental hospital; depressives and neurotics under the care of psychiatrists as outpatients; patients in a general hospital who showed symptoms of depression or exhibited neurotic manifestations superimposed on physical diseases and patients who had senile dementia, anxiety or depression.

Trazodone was administered orally in capsule form in the following dosages:

Case	Dosage, mg/day
Schizophrenia	300–400
Neurosis	30–250
Senile patients	30– 70
Depressives	200–300

Duration of therapy was from 42 to 180 days.

Table I. Therapeutic effects of trazodone

Diagnosis	Number of cases	Number of effective cases (excellent and fair)	Rate of effectiveness, %
Schizophrenia	12	4	33.3
Depression	8	6	75.0
Neurosis	38	20	52.6
Senility	4	2	50.0
Total	62	32	51.6

Therapeutic effects of trazodone are shown in table I.

There was a transient calming effect in schizophrenics. A mild increase of volition was observed along with a stabilizing action on emotions. Antidepressant and stabilizing effects were also noted in depressed patients.

Among neurotics, especially those suffering from anxiety neurosis responded favourably to trazodone. The negative emotional aspects concerning their anxiety experiences were lessened and their feelings of well being were increased. In a few patients euphoric states were observed.

These emotional states became stabilized in the course of treatment not merely by the tranquilizing action of the drug, but also by an increase of volition.

Senile patients with mild depressive psychopathological symptoms superimposed on organic changes such as cerebral arteriosclerosis attained an elevation of mood and a feeling of stability from relatively smaller dosages of trazodone shortly after administration of the drug, i. e. within 3–4 days.

Small dosages of trazodone provided relief to subjects suffering from anxiety with tension.

Trazodone, however, even in a large dosage, was shown to be ineffective in patients exhibiting lack of spontaneity (which is the fundamental disturbance of schizophrenics) and in severe schizophrenics.

It was not possible to block cyclothymic depression, to prevent the recurrence of depression and/or to shorten its duration.

The most favorable results were obtained in cases of pre-senile depression, or involutional melancholia.

In our clinical studies, trazodone was ineffective in hysteria and chronic character neurosis. Exacerbation of symptoms, such as instability, irritability and insomnia, was noted in 6 out of 8 cases of hysteria.

On the basis of these observations, the clinical effects of trazodone can be described as quick and short-acting and can be characterized as 'Vitale Erhebung' or 'Antriebssteigerung'. Trazodone, we believe, can safely be employed in the treatment of outpatients in conjunction with psychotherapy, because its clinical sedative effects is stronger than that of diazepam, and its side-effects are almost negligible.

Summary

1. A mild increase of volition and a stabilizing action on emotions in schizophrenics.
2. Anti-depressive and stabilizing effects in depressed patients.
3. A tranquilizing effect in anxiety neurotics: (a) decrease of negative emotions; (b) increase in feeling of happiness; (c) appearance of euphoric states.
4. Ineffective in severe schizophrenics.
5. Ineffective in hysterical and character neurotics.
6. Exacerbation of symptoms (instability, irritability and insomnia) in hysterical neurosis.
7. Rather quick onset of action and short-lasting effect.
8. Negligible side effects with daily doses of less than 400 mg.

Author's address: Dr. Takashi Shibahara, Director, Department of Psychiatry, Kyoto First Red Cross Hospital, *Kyoto* (Japan)

Trazodone. Mod. Probl. Pharmacopsychiat., vol. 9, pp. 176–181,
ed. Th. A. Ban, Montreal, Que., and B. Silvestrini, Rome (Karger, Basel 1974)

Clinical Effect of Intravenous Trazodone Administration in Severe Depression

F. Pariante

Psychiatric Hospital of Volterra, Pisa

In our clinical comparisons of trazodone versus imipramine employing the double-blind crossover method, we found that trazodone, administered orally, exerts significant therapeutic effects in severe depression. In particular, there was significant improvement in symptoms of depressed mood, interest in work and activities, and mental and motor retardation as assessed by the Hamilton Rating Scale for Depression (HAM). Moreover, there were no major undesirable side effects, and good tolerance of trazodone was observed in all the patients treated orally.

In an open and more extensive clinical trial trazodone was administered i. v. to 20 subjects admitted mainly for depressive illness.

Method

Subject

Of the 20 patients studied there were 13 (6 men and 7 women) with endogenous or endoreactive depression, 4 women with reactive depression, and 1 male and 1 female with obsessive-phobic neurosis. One female with Cotard's syndrome was included in the study. These patients ranged in age from 24 to 72 years with an average of 51.95 years of age (table I).

Procedure

After a three-day, placebo washout, 100–200 mg of trazodone in a 200 ml saline solution were administered i. v. twice or three times daily. Each infusion lasted nearly 2 h. The length of treatment (7 to 21 days) and the total doses (table I) were established on the basis of clinical evaluation.

Table I

Case No.	Sex	Age, years	Diagnosis	Mean daily dose, mg	Time of treatment, days	First effect, days	Clinical findings
1	F	51	reactive depression	300	15	7	normalized
2	F	63	endogenous depression	250	21	15	normalized
3	F	70	endogenous depression	250	15	7	improvement
4	M	34	endoreact. depression	300	21	7	normalized
5	M	66	endogenous depression	300	21	7	normalized
6	F	70	endogenous depression	250	15	7	improvement
7	F	24	reactive depression	400	15	7	normalized
8	F	72	endogenous depression	300	7	–	deteriorated
9	F	44	reactive depression	500	15	7	normalized
10	F	59	endogenous depression	500	15	7	normalized
11	M	53	endogenous depression	300	15	7	normalized
12	M	40	endogenous depression	300	15	7	normalized
13	M	46	endogenous depression	300	15	7	normalized
14	F	38	obsessive neurosis	400	7	–	no change
15	M	33	obsessive neurosis	400	21	15	improvement
16	F	63	Cotard's syndrome	250	21	–	no change
17	F	34	endogenous depression	500	11	5	normalized
18	F	45	reactive depression	300	9	6	normalized
19	F	72	endogenous depression	400	10	–	no change
20	M	62	endogenous depression	500	16	7	improvement

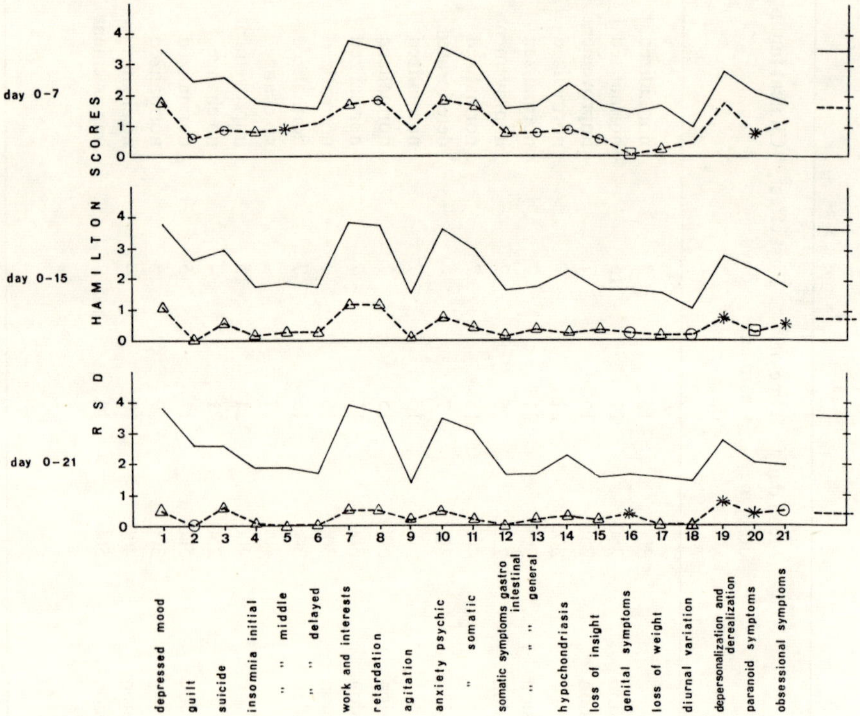

Fig. 1. Clinical changes during i. v. treatment with trazodone (Hamilton Rating Scale for Depression). — = Before; --- = after; △ = $p < 0.001$; ○ = $p < 0.01$; □ = $p < 0.02$; ★ = $p < 0.05$.

The i. v. administration lasted until definite improvement, substantiated by both clinical observation and rating scale scores, was obtained. Treatment was carried on by oral administration. Table I shows the time of the treatment and the mean daily dose.

Therapeutic activity was assessed by two observers on the basis of continuous clinical observations and also through analysis of scores on the HAM and the Brief Psychiatric Rating Scale (BPRS) of Overall and Gorham. These results were completed before treatment began and on the 7th, 15th and 21st day of treatment. Figures 1 and 2 illustrate the mean pretreatment scores in comparison with scores obtained at each of the later rating periods. The significance of the difference is also reported in figures 1 and 2.

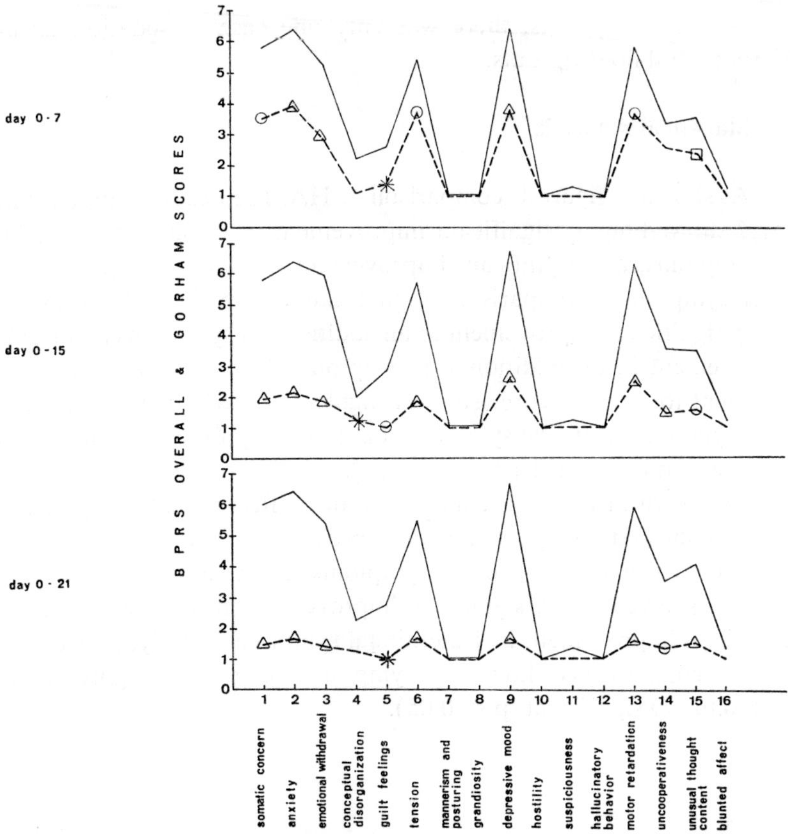

Fig. 2. Clinical changes during i. v. treatment with trazodone (Brief Psychiatric Rating Scale of Overall and Gorham scores). — = Before; - - - = after; △ = $p < 0.001$; ○ = $p < 0.01$; □ = $p < 0.02$; ☆ = $p < 0.05$.

Results

Clinical Findings

The clinical findings are summarized in table I. 12 of the patients showed complete recovery, 4 improved significantly, while 4 patients (1 obsessive neurosis, 1 Cotard's syndrome and 1 endogenous depression) remained unchanged, and 1 other patient (endogenous depression) deteriorated over the course of treatment.

In 14 of the patients the first positive effects were observed after 5 to 7 days of treatment.

As for side effects, there was only one case of sedation during the infusions and no drop-outs.

Statistical Analysis

As shown in figure 1, comparison of HAM scores from pretreatment to day 7 showed highly significant improvement ($p < 0.001$ to $p < 0.01$) in 13 symptoms, and significant improvement ($p < 0.01$ to $p < 0.05$) in 3 other symptoms. Comparison of pretreatment to day 15 scores showed highly significant improvement in an additional 5 symptoms and significant improvement in an additional 2 symptoms. Finally, comparison of pretreatment to day 21 scores showed highly significant improvement in one more symptom, with one symptom going from highly significant ($p < 0.02$) to somewhat less significant ($p < 0.05$).

As shown in figure 2, comparison of BPRS scores from pretreatment to day 7 showed highly significant improvement in 6 symptoms and significant improvement in 2 other symptoms. Pretreatment to day 15 comparisons showed highly significant improvement in 3 more symptoms and significant improvement in 1 additional symptom. Finally, pretreatment to day 21 comparisons showed 1 symptom going from highly significant ($p < 0.02$) to significant ($p < 0.05$).

Conclusion

Present findings, in accordance with our previous investigations, suggest that trazodone is effective in depressed mood and anxiety.

By the i. v. administration, with the doses employed by us, the therapeutic effect appears to be rapid and selective on the peculiar symptoms of the depressive syndrome, i. e. depressive mood, feeling of guilt, suicidal thoughts, anxiety, tension, emotional withdrawal, motor retardation, decreased mental productivity, decreased productivity in the work and interests, uncooperativeness, insomnia, somatic concern and hypocondriasis. Other symptoms such as unusual thoughts and agitation, are positively affected at a later time.

These observations also confirm that trazodone does not have a neuroleptic activity, a sedative effect being observed only during i. v. administration.

In conclusion, on the basis of our data, trazodone appears to be highly effective in endogenous and reactive depression.

Reference

PARIANTE, F.: Un nuovo antidepressivo: il Trazodone, valutazione della sua attività con studio double-blind con cross-over. Riv. Neuropsichiat. *17:* 1–19 (1971).

Author's address: F. PARIANTE, Ph. D., Psychiatric Hospital of Volterra, *Pisa* (Italy)

Trazodone. Mod. Probl. Pharmacopsychiat., vol. 9, pp. 182–189,
ed. Th. A. Ban, Montreal, Que., and B. Silvestrini, Rome (Karger, Basel 1974)

Polygraphic Study of the All-Night Sleep Pattern in Neurotic and Depressed Patients Treated with Trazodone

A. Muratorio, C. Maggini, G. Coccagna and M. Guazzelli

Istituto di Clinica Psichiatrica, Università di Pisa,
II Clinica Malattie nervose e mentali, Università di Pisa,
Clinica Malattie nervose e mentali, Università di Bologna, Bologna

Polygraphic sleep pattern investigations of normals, neurotics and psychotics are a valid and objective parameter to recognize and assess important characteristics of a new psychoactive compound [Itil, 1972; Itil *et al.*, 1968; Bedarida *et al.*, 1969; Maggini *et al.*, 1969 a, b].

The hypothesis that different psychopathological syndromes are associated with specific modifications of the sleep pattern is supported by psychopharmacological experiments [Sarteschi *et al.*, 1969; Maggini *et al.*, 1969 a, b; Castrogiovanni *et al.*, 1971].

Previous studies have shown that drug-induced changes of the sleep EEG pattern are correlated with changes of the psychopathological picture [Muratorio and Maggini, 1969; Maggini *et al.*, 1969 a, b].

This work deals with some preliminary data obtained in a multicenter study not yet completed at the time of publication of this volume. In this study the EEG changes, induced by trazodone on the sleep of neurotic and depressed patients were investigated during three different experimental conditions: (a) single dose administration; (b) pilot study; (c) controlled, double-blind clinical trial. The material and method of these experiments are reported in detail (table I).

Table I. Experimental designs

	Treatment		Number of subjects	Age, years	Sex	Diagnosis	Time of recording, days		
	drug	dose, mg/day					before treatment	during treatment	after treatment
Single dose	trazodone	50	4	40.5	M	psychoneurosis	2nd, 3rd	4th, 5th, 6th	7th, 8th
Pilot open study	trazodone	300–600	6	49.0	M	5 endogenous depressions, 1 psychoneurosis	2nd	6th, 10th, 14th	
Controlled double-blind trial	trazodone	250–500	5	59.1	F	endogenous depression	2nd	3rd, 7th	
	imipramine	75–150	3[1]	52.0	F			14th	

1 As the study for this preliminary report was not yet concluded we took from the EEG Laboratory data bank of the Psychiatric Clinic of Pisa 7 additional endogenous depressive patients previously treated with imipramine.

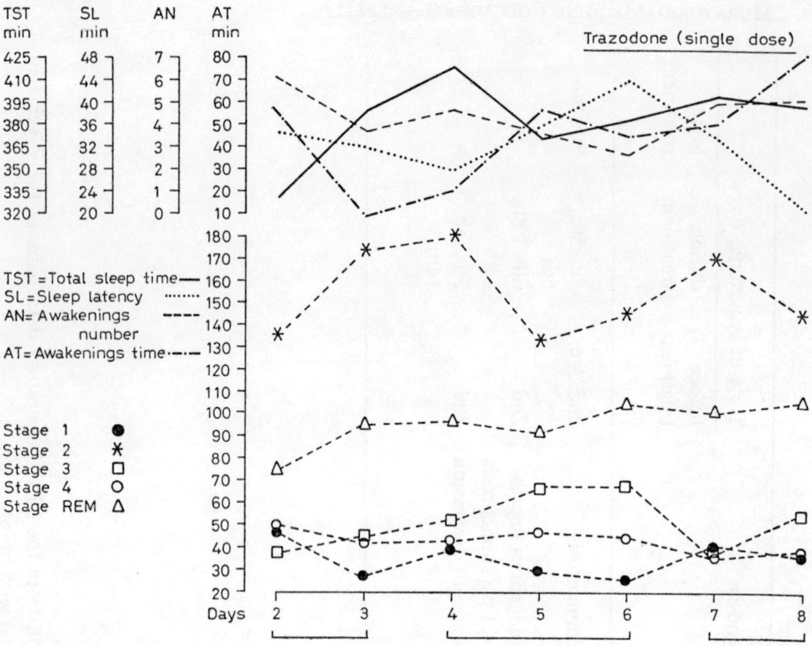
TST min
SL min
AN
AT min
Trazodone (single dose)
TST = Total sleep time
SL = Sleep latency
AN = Awakenings number
AT = Awakenings time
Stage 1
Stage 2
Stage 3
Stage 4
Stage REM
Days

Fig. 1

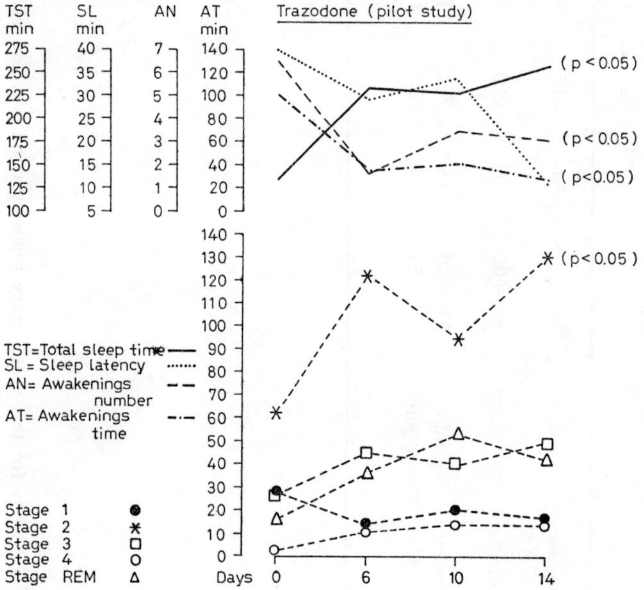
TST min
SL min
AN
AT min
Trazodone (pilot study)
(p < 0.05)
(p < 0.05)
(p<0.05)
(p< 0.05)
TST=Total sleep time
SL = Sleep latency
AN= Awakenings number
AT= Awakenings time
Stage 1
Stage 2
Stage 3
Stage 4
Stage REM
Days

Fig. 2

A. Single Dose

This trial was set up in order to ascertain the sleep-inducing properties of trazodone and to check whether a single administration of this drug induces significant changes of the sleep pattern which could allow for a first screening of the compound.

In these patients the basal recordings were characterized by a normal sleep time with a slight increase in sleep latency; the other sleep parameters, the traditional stages, were very close to normal values. The patients had mild neurotic symptoms and could be considered good sleepers. In these subjects administration of 50 mg of trazodone at night did not induce meaningful changes in the sleep pattern (fig. 1). Similar results were obtained in normals and in neurotic good sleepers with oxazepam, although this drug showed eupnic properties in neurotics with disturbed sleep (MURATORIO and MAGGINI, 1967].

B. Pilot Study

The basal sleep of these subjects was characterized by a decrease of total sleep time, an increase of sleep latency and of the number and duration of awake periods. Stages 1 and 2 were increased, whereas stages 3 and 4 and REM were reduced.

During trazodone treatment the total sleep time and the number and duration of awakenings were significantly modified. Analysis of variance showed a significant ($p < 0.05$) increase in total sleep time and a significant decrease in the number and duration of awakenings ($p < 0.05$). Moreover, trazodone induces a significant increase of stage 2 sleep ($p < 0.05$) due to the increase of total sleep time and a decrease of stage 1 due to the reduction of the number of awake periods. Stage 3, although not significantly, was clearly increased (fig. 2, table II).

Similar results were obtained by discriminant analysis (fig. 3). Stage 4, which is typically increased by tricyclic antidepressant drugs, was not modified by trazodone. These data are in agreement with the clinical ratings and seem to suggest that trazodone may be slightly closer to the antianxiety benzodiazepines than to the antidepressant tricyclic compounds.

C. Controlled Double-Blind Clinical Trial

The basal EEGs showed the typical sleep pattern of endogenous depression (fig. 4). Trazodone treatment produced an increase of stage 3

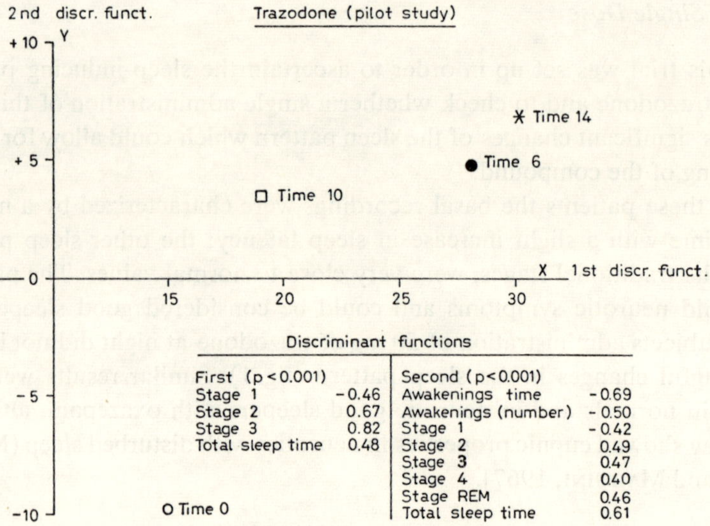
2nd discr. funct.
Y
Trazodone (pilot study)
+10
+5
0
-5
-10
15
20
25
30
X 1st discr. funct.
Time 14
Time 6
Time 10
Time 0
Discriminant functions
First (p < 0.001)
Stage 1 -0.46
Stage 2 0.67
Stage 3 0.82
Total sleep time 0.48
Second (p < 0.001)
Awakenings time -0.69
Awakenings (number) -0.50
Stage 1 -0.42
Stage 2 0.49
Stage 3 0.47
Stage 4 0.40
Stage REM 0.46
Total sleep time 0.61

Fig. 3

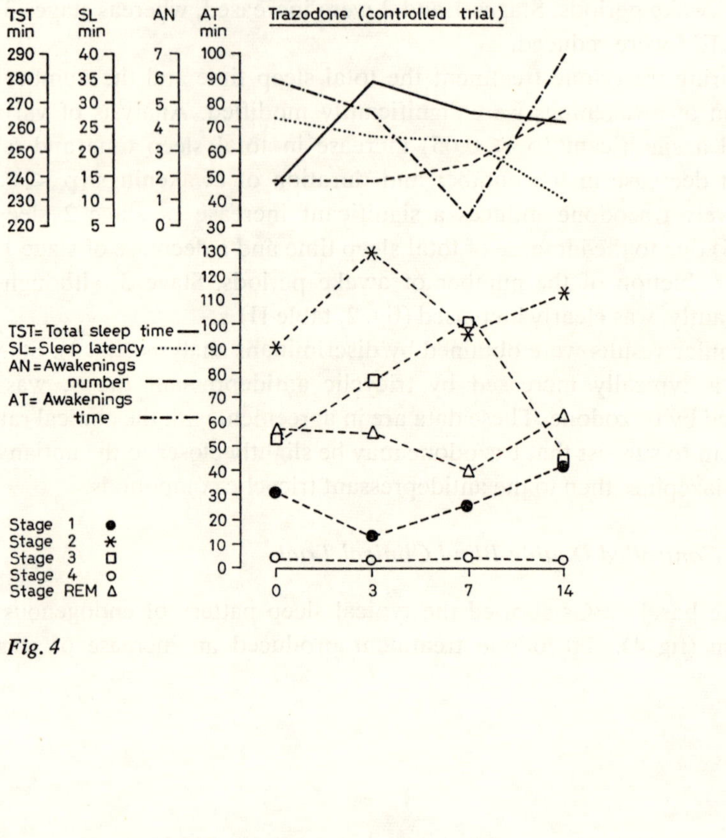
TST min
SL min
AN
AT min
Trazodone (controlled trial)
TST=Total sleep time
SL=Sleep latency
AN=Awakenings number
AT=Awakenings time
Stage 1
Stage 2
Stage 3
Stage 4
Stage REM
0
3
7
14

Fig. 4

Table II. Effects of trazodone (pilot study) on the sleep stages (% TST)

	Basal recording	Days of treatment			Analysis of variance	
		6th	10th	14th	F ratio	p
Stage 1	21.44	7.08	8.73	6.11	10.58	0.01
Stage 2	46.55	50.69	43.60	51.19	0.58	–
Stage 3	19.71	19.41	20.42	20.34	0.02	–
Stage 4	1.38	6.85	8.59	5.56	0.84	–
Stage REM	11.05	15.93	18.62	16.76	0.32	–

Table III. Effects of trazodone (controlled trial) on the sleep stages (% TST)

	Basal recording	Days of treatment			Analysis of variance	
		3rd	7th	14th	F ratio	p
Stage 1	14.51	6.89	9.90	15.48	1.02	–
Stage 2	43.36	41.88	36.44	42.92	0.18	–
Stage 3	21.03	29.60	36.86	18.38	3.48	0.04
Stage 4	2.15	0.94	1.31	1.67	0.16	–
Stage REM	18.92	20.68	15.47	21.53	0.23	–

Table IV. Effects of imipramine on the sleep stages (% TST)

	Basal recording	Days of treatment			Analysis of variance	
		3rd	7th	14th	F ratio	p
Stage 1	28.46	23.06	18.62	19.69	0.81	–
Stage 2	40.38	47.17	44.35	48.42	0.85	–
Stage 3	11.45	13.11	19.14	13.22	1.52	–
Stage 4	1.22	4.28	7.53	7.60	3.20	0.03
Stage REM	18.04	12.34	10.32	11.04	1.51	–

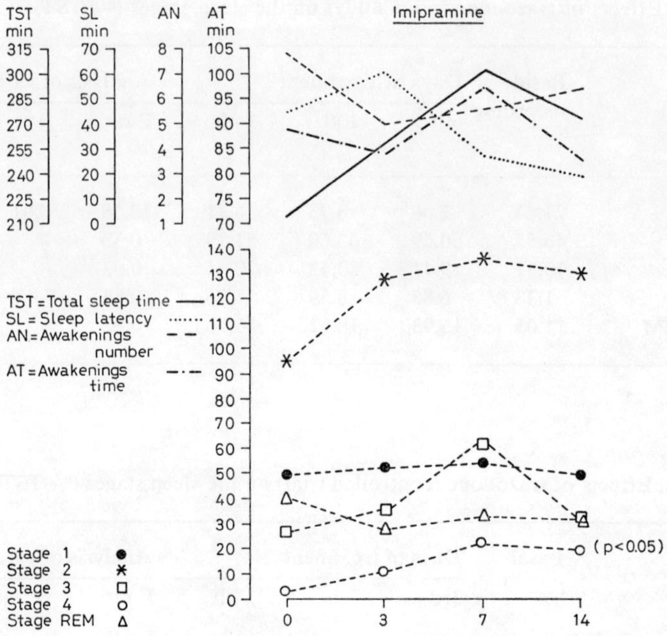

Fig. 5

in percent of total sleep time (table III), whereas in the imipramine treated group there was a typical increase of stage 4 (fig. 5, table IV). The effect of trazodone, limited to an increase of stage 3, seems to be in this trial less broad than in the pilot study where total sleep time, number and duration of awakenings and stages 1 and 2, were also modified.

It was also noted that whereas the clinical and polygraphic changes induced by trazodone appeared rapidly at the beginning of treatment, the effects of imipramine on the depressive symptoms, and on the sleep pattern, appeared at later times.

In conclusion:

1. Trazodone in a single small dose does not appear to have any sleep-inducing properties in neurotic good sleepers.

2. On the basis of this polygraphic investigation trazodone does not seem to be similar to tricyclic antidepressant compounds, since changes on sleep patterns in depressed patients appear to be different from the ones

produced by other antidepressants. In particular, we did not observe the typical increase of stage 4 as induced by tricyclic drugs.

3. Trazodone in the most commonly administered dose has often shown in depressed patients an effect similar, to a certain extent, to that produced by anti-anxiety drugs. Such an effect is characterized by a marked increase of total sleep time, caused by a decrease of the number of awake periods, leading to a better distribution of sleep stages (i. e. a decrease of stage 1 and an increase of stage 2). Nevertheless, during trazodone treatment we did not observe any changes during the REM stage similar to those reported during benzodiazepine treatment.

References

Bedarida, D.; Maggini, C.; Riccioni, R.; Castrogiovanni, P. e Cassano, G. B.: Valutazione dell'azione ansiolitica ed euipnica di un nuovo derivato benzodiazepinico (ER 115). Indagine clinico-poligrafica. Atti II Riun. Naz. Soc. Ist. Neuropsicofarmacol. Tirrenia, Pisa 1969.

Castrogiovanni, P.; Placidi, G. F.; Maggini, C.; Ghetti, B., and Cassano, G. B.: Clinical investigation of doxepin in depressed patients. Pilot open study, controlled double-blind trial versus imipramine and all-night polygraphic study. Pharmakopsychiat. Neuro-Psychopharm. *4:* 170–181 (1971).

Itil, T. M.: Quantitative pharmaco-electroencephalography, a new method in drug screening. Proc. 8th Ann. Meet. Drug Information Ass., New York 1972.

Itil, T. M.; Shapiro, D., and Fink, M.: Differentiation of psychotropic drugs by quantitative EEG analysis. Agressologia *9:* 267–280 (1968).

Maggini, C.; Gallevi, M.; Conti, L.; Placidi, S. F. e Castrogiovanni, P.: Impiego dell'indagine poligrafica del sonno nello studio delle caratteristiche di un nuovo psicofarmaco (AF 1161). Boll. Soc. Med. Chir. Pisa *4:* 294–305 (1969 a).

Maggini, C.; Murri, L., and Sacchetti, G.: Evaluation of the effectiveness of Temazepam on the insomnia of patients with neurosis and endogenous depression. Arzneimittelforsch. *19:* 1647–1652 (1969 b).

Muratorio, A. e Maggini, C.: Studio poligrafico del sonno notturno in soggetti normali e psiconevrotici trattati con oxazepam. Rass. Studi psichiat. *56:* 654–669 (1967).

Muratorio, A. e Maggini, C.: Psicofarmaci e sonno. Neopsichiatria *35:* 33–133 (1969).

Sarteschi, P.; Cassano, G. B., and Maggini, C.: Polygraphic study of all-night sleep in Schizophrenics treated with thioridazine. Symp. Pharmacological and Clinical Aspects of Psychotropic Drug Therapy, Mosca 1969.

Author's address: Dr. A. Muratorio, II Clinica Malattie nervose e mentali Università di Pisa, *Pisa* (Italy)

Third Clinical Session

Chairman: A. Villeneuve

Trazodone. Mod. Probl. Pharmacopsychiat., vol. 9, pp. 190–198,
ed. Th. A. Ban, Montreal, Que., and B. Silvestrini, Rome (Karger, Basel 1974)

Trazodone versus Desipramine: A Double-Blind Study on the Rapidity of the Antidepressive Effect

A. Agnoli, M. Piccione, M. Casacchia and C. Fazio

Department of Neurology and Psychiatry, University of Rome, Rome

The antidepressive drugs belong to the tricyclic and MAO-inhibitor groups. Although these drugs have satisfactory therapeutic properties, they also produce a variety of side-effects. Consequently, further research for drugs having equal or higher antidepressive activity but only minor side-effects, is justified.

Trazodone belongs to a new chemical group with unusual pharmacological effects: on the basis of pharmacological findings a potential usefulness of the drug as an antidepressant has been postulated [1].

The aim of this work is not to reevaluate the antidepressive action of the drug [2] but to report on a double-blind study comparing the rapidity of action of the antidepressive effects of trazodone with that of desipramine (DMI).

Material and Design of the Trial

Subjects

30 patients were selected and divided into two equal groups at random. They were all between 21 and 67 years of age (average 40.1); 6 males and 24 females. The types of depression were as follows:

Endogenous depression	26
Endoreactive depression	1
Reactive depression	2
Involutive depression	1

Procedure

The degree of severity of the depressive syndrome and the changes in the symptoms during therapy were evaluated by two methods: the Hamilton Rating Scale for Depression (HAM) and the Rapid Index of Psychopharmacological Efficiency (RIPE).

The first [3], which is well known, needs no explanation (21 items were considered). The second [4] is a method used to evaluate the rapidity of action of a psychoactive drug (4 items were considered): (a) the main symptoms of the depression, (b) anxiety, (c) hypochondriasis, (d) disturbances of ideation. 20 items were mentioned at five different levels, with a score ranging from 0 to 4 as follows: 0 = no symptoms; 1 = light; 2 = medium; 3 = severe; 4 = very severe.

The rating scales were completed before treatment, on the third day of therapy, on the 7th day and at the end of treatment (15th day). The patients were randomly assigned to groups A and B. The drugs were given in identical capsule form following a double-blind design. Each capsule contained trazodone 100 mg and DMI 25 mg.

The dosage regime for both products was as follows:

Treatment was started with two capsules per day for two days, then one capsule was added per day for the next three days. By the 14th day 5 capsules were given, or 6 in severe cases.

All patients who presented liver, heart, renal or neurological alterations before therapy were excluded. Both before and during therapy the usual hematochemical tests were carried out as well as an EEG. No other drugs were used except for pentobarbital (0.1 g in the evening) or a mild tranquilizer (diazepam 5 mg t. i. d.).

Results

The changes in total score of the RIPE scale for the two groups are shown in figure 1: the average score obtained is on the ordinate and the times of examination on the abscissa.

This figure shows that the patients treated with trazodone had a higher score before treatment than those on DMI. However, on the 3rd and 5th day this finding was reversed, whereas on the 7th and 14th day the patients on trazodone had a higher score than those on DMI.

If one compares the scores in relation to time, both groups appear very much the same. Thus, on the 14th day the score for the trazodone-treated group had decreased 84.2 % and the DMI group 85 % from pretreatment levels.

Figure 2 shows the variation of scores on the Hamilton scale for the two groups. The results confirm our previous observations. The decreases in percentage on the 14th day in the trazodone-treated group was 80 % and in the DMI group 79 %.

A statistical analysis of the total and partial scores in the two scales,

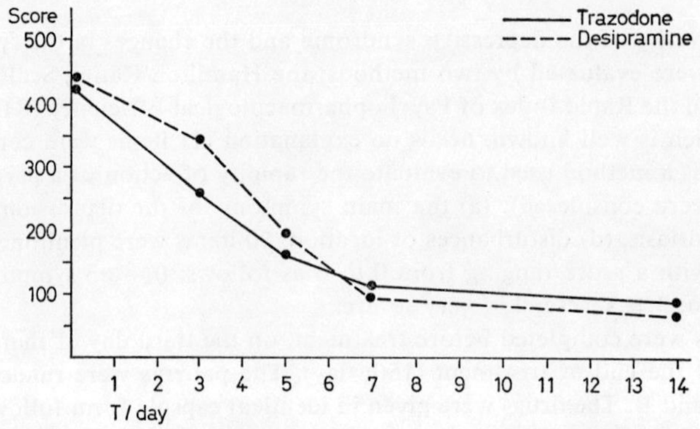

Fig. 1. Rapid Index of Psychopharmacological Efficiency (RIPE). Variations of the total score during the treatment. Comparison of the effect of the two drugs.

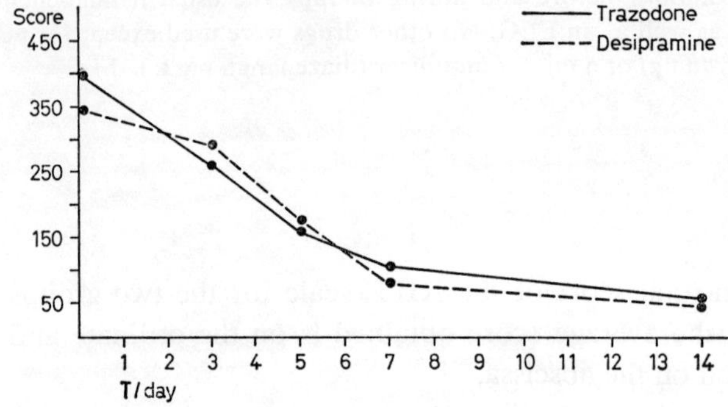

Fig. 2. Hamilton Rating Scale for Depression (HAM). Variations of the total score during the treatment. Comparison of the effect of the two drugs.

comparing the scores before treatment, with scores on the 3rd day and at the end of treatment, showed the following:

1. Analysis of variance of the average initial scores for each item on the Hamilton scale did not show any significant variation between the subjects treated with trazodone and those treated with desipramine. There was, therefore, no heterogeneity in the basal data used in this study.

2. Analysis of covariance (total final scores for each item on the Hamilton scale) showed that on the 3rd day there was a significant difference only

Table I. Evaluation of the clinical symptoms with the HAM (21 items)

Hamilton scale	Covariance analysis		Student's t-test for coupled data					
			trazodone			desipramine		
	'F'	p	n	%	p	n	%	p
0→3								
Total score	1.695	n. s.	15	31	<0.001	14	17	n. s.
Suicide	0.220	n. s.	8	29	<0.05	8	19	n. s.
Retardation	1.647	n. s.	15	33	<0.02	11	5.5	n. s.
Agitation	2.661	n. s.	11	67	<0.001	9	31	n. s.
Anxiety psychic	4.107	n. s.	8	46	<0.01	10	+15	n. s.
Anxiety somatic	11.034	< 0.01	8	67	<0.02	10	+22	n. s.
Genital symptoms	5.841	< 0.05	11	17	n. s.	8	+16	n. s.
Loss of weight	3.441	n. s.	14	5	n. s.	9	40	< 0.05
0→7								
Hypochondriasis	0.562	n. s.	7	37	n. s.	10	65	< 0.001
0→14								
Hypochondriasis	0.051	n. s.	6	56	n. s.	10	71	< 0.001

The covariance analysis refers to the scores obtained during trazodone and desipramine treatment. The t-test refers to the scores obtained during the same treatment, at different times. Only the items in which a significant activity was observed are reported.

between somatic anxiety and genital symptoms in favour of trazodone (table I). A comparison of the other items was not significant. On the 7th and 14 th day there was no significant difference between trazodone and DMI. Analysis of the data obtained on the RIPE scale was not significant (tables II–IV).

3. The analyses of the coupled data gave the following results: in the different items of the HAM only some subjects of the trazodone treated group were favourably influenced (significant $p < 0.001$).

On the 3rd day significant results as compared to pretreatment scores were obtained in these items: suicide, retardation, agitation, psychic and somatic anxiety (table I).

On the 7th and 14th day, the hypochondriasis was favourably influenced by trazodone, as opposed to DMI. All other symptoms were equally and significantly influenced.

Table II. Evaluation of the clinical symptoms with the RIPE

RIPE 0→3	Covariance analysis		Student's t-test for coupled data					
			trazodone			desipramine		
	'F'	p	n	%	p	n	%	p
Total score	1.170	n. s.	15	39	<0.001	14	22	< 0.05
Typical symptoms of depression	0.567	n. s.	15	36	<0.001	14	29	< 0.001
Anxiety	3.061	n. s.	11	56	<0.01	11	12	n. s.
Hypochondriasis	2.264	n. s.	10	46	<0.05	13	5	n. s.

The covariance analysis refers to the scores obtained during trazodone and desipramine treatment. The t-test refers to the scores obtained during the same treatment, at different times. Only the items in which a significant activity was observed are reported.

The RIPE scale showed lesser differences: in fact, on the 3rd day all the items were equally and significantly influenced by both drugs, with the exception of anxiety and hypochondriasis, which were only influenced by trazodone (table II). On the 7th and 14th day the pharmacological effects were the same for both drugs (table III, IV).

4. The reduced percentages between the initial points and those on the 3rd day allowed us to run a G test for each item on the Hamilton and RIPE scales. The criteria adopted in each case in relation to the percent reduction were as follows: worse; up to 10% improvement; 11–40% improvement; over 40% improvement.

The G test showed a significant difference in favour of trazodone for the following items: psychic anxiety ($p<0.05$); somatic anxiety ($p<0.02$); genital symptoms ($p<0.05$) on the Hamilton scale. In the RIPE 'anxiety' symptoms: $p<0.02$.

The percentual variations between pretreatment scores and day 3, as calculated for all items on the Hamilton scale, are summarized in table V and VI.

We can state that whereas trazodone has a favourable influence and works rapidly in the anxiety nucleus, the initial action of DMI is less specific.

Table III. Evaluation of the clinical symptoms with the RIPE

RIPE 0→7	Covariance analysis		Student's t-test for coupled data					
			trazodone			desipramine		
	'F'	p	n	%	p	n	%	p
Total score	0.168	n. s.	15	76	<0.001	14	78	< 0.001
Typical symptoms of depression	0	n. s.	15	80	<0.001	14	80	< 0.001
Anxiety	0.235	n. s.	11	77	<0.001	9	73	< 0.01
Hypochondriasis	1.350	n. s.	10	58	<0.02	13	82	< 0.001

The covariance analysis refers to the scores obtained during trazodone and desipramine treatment. The t-test refers to the scores obtained during the same treatment, at different times. Only the items in which a significant activity was observed are reported.

The antidepressive effect of the two drugs is similar in that both the depressed mood and suicide are equally influenced. While DMI worsens the anxiety symptoms (+22%), trazodone does not worsen any symptoms.

Finally, on the basis of the percentage of improvement of those symptoms that are most influenced on the third day, it is possible to state that trazodone has a better effect on the depressive nucleus than DMI.

The above data also suggest a rapidity of action as per evaluation on the third day of treatment. Side-effects were evaluated by a proper side-effect RS. Only one case of glaucoma was noted in a patient treated with DMI, while no side-effects were noted in patients treated with trazodone.

The above data show that in all cases treated there was a favourable response in the treatment of the depressive symptoms.

Discussion

An examination of the results leads to the following conclusions:

1. The two groups of patients studied were not heterogeneous; they can be considered homogeneous.

2. The depressive symptoms' improvement was shown on the third day

Table IV. Evaluation of the clinical with the RIPE

RIPE 0→14	Covariance analysis		Student's t-test for coupled data					
			trazodone			desipramine		
	'F'	p	n	%	p	n	%	p
Total score	0.298	n. s.	15	80	<0.001	14	80	< 0.001
Typical symptoms of depression	0.044	n. s.	15	83	<0.001	14	87	< 0.001
Anxiety	0.566	n. s.	11	77	<0.001	9	77	< 0.01
Hypochondriasis	0.629	n. s.	10	66	<0.01	13	82	< 0.001

The covariance analysis refers to the scores obtained during trazodone and desipramine treatment. The t-test refers to the scores obtained during the same treatment, at different times. Only the items in which a significant activity was observed are reported.

Table V. HAM results on the third day of the treatment

Symptoms improved (decreasing order) Trazodone	Desipramine
Agitation and anxiety somatic	insomnia, initial
Insomnia	guilt
Initial	loss of weight
Delayed	insomnia delayed
Anxiety psychic	agitation
Insomnia middle	
Guilt	
Depressed mood	*depressed mood*
Retardation	somatic general symptoms
Suicide	*suicide*
Somatic symptoms	somatic symptoms
Works and interests	hypochondriasis
Symptoms worsened	
None	anxiety psychic
	anxiety somatic
	genital symptoms

Table VI. HAM symptoms on the third day of the treatment (% variation regarding pretreatment scores)

	Trazodone	Desipramine
Depressed mood	–39.4	–27.7
Suicide	–29.4	–19.0
Insomnia, delayed	–50.0	–34.8
Work and interests	–21.7	– 7.8
Agitation	–66.6	–30.7
Anxiety	–66.6	+22

of treatment; somatic anxiety and genital symptoms were more influenced by trazodone than by DMI. The other symptoms were equally and significantly influenced, and therefore both treatments were equally active in the same period. Trazodone has, however, a faster and better action on anxiety symptoms.

3. When we consider the results obtained referring to a single treatment, the following conclusions can be drawn. The HAM on the third day showed that although some items reacted favourably to trazodone therapy, no significant results were observed with DMI. On the 7th and 14 th day the drugs showed equal activity. The RIPE scale gave similar results. We can therefore conclude that trazodone has a more rapid action than DMI on some items.

4. If we consider those symptoms which are most significantly influenced by the treatment, we observe that both with the HAM and with the RIPE scale, the anxiety nucleus and the genital symptoms are those which are most influenced on the third day by trazodone.

If we consider in the decreasing order the symptoms which are most influenced, we can see that trazodone has a rapid anxiolytic effect while DMI makes the anxiety nucleus worse (+22 %).

The depressive state and suicidal ideas are equally influenced in the same time period, even if trazodone seems to be more active (10–15 % more than DMI).

In conclusion, trazodone has an antidepressive effect which is equally rapid and slightly more potent than DMI. It has a very rapid anxiolytic effect which is not obtained with DMI which, on the other hand, worsens the anxiety nucleus.

References

1 Silvestrini, B.; Cioli, V.; Burberi, S., and Catanese, B.: Pharmacological properties of AF 1161, a new psychotropic drug. Int. J. Neuropharmacol. *7:* 587–589 (1968).

2 de Gregorio, M. and Dionisio, A.: A controlled chimical study of a new antidepressant (Trazodone). Panminerva med. *23:* 1–2, 27–30 (1971).

3 Hamilton, M.: A rating scale for depression. J. Neurol. Neurosurg. Psychiatr. *23:* 56–62 (1960).

4 Capitanucci, P.; de Gregorio, M. e Dall'Aglio, E.: L'indice rapido di efficacia farmacologica. Formula A: per lo Studio clinico dei farmaci antidepressivi. Med. Psicosom. *13:* 3–12 (1968).

Authors' address: A. Agnoli, M. Piccione, M. Casacchia and C. Facio, Department of Neurology and Psychiatry, University of Rome, *Rome* (Italy)

Trazodone. Mod. Probl. Pharmacopsychiat., vol. 9, pp. 199–204,
ed. Th. A. Ban, Montreal, Que., and B. Silvestrini, Rome (Karger, Basel 1974)

Clinical Evaluation of Trazodone in the Treatment of Depression

G. B. CASSANO, P. CASTROGIOVANNI and L. CONTI

Psychiatric Clinic, University of Pisa, Pisa

Introduction

Trazodone, 2-(N-[m-chlorophenyl]-piperazino)-propyl-s-triazolo-(4,3-a)pyridine-3-one, is a new psychotropic drug with a spectrum of pharmacological activity unlike that of any known drug [SILVESTRINI *et al.* 1968]. Previous clinical investigations have suggested its possible use in various psychopathological conditions [CONTI *et al.*, 1969; DE GREGORIO and DIONISIO, 1969; 1971].

In this paper the results of three clinical trials are reported, i. e., a pilot study, a controlled double-blind trial and a polygraphic all-night sleep investigation. They were performed at the Psychiatric Clinic in Pisa.

Methods

In the *pilot study* 20 inpatients (mean age 55; 10 males and 10 females) with primarily depressive and anxiety symptoms (7 retarded, 6 anxious, 4 paranoid depressions and 3 psychoneurosis) were admitted to the trial.

After a 3 to 5-day placebo washout, trazodone was given at 'non-fixed' doses corresponding to a mean of 300 mg/day in the first two days, 400 mg/day from 2 to 6, 500 mg/day from 6 to 10 and 600 mg/day from 10 to 14 days.

In the *controlled study,* 31 female inpatients with a mean age of 54 (22 endogenous and 9 endoreactive depressions) were admitted to a 'between-groups' double-blind trial.

After a 3 to 5-day placebo treatment, imipramine or trazodone were given at random. Trazodone was first given at the mean dose of 354 mg/day, reaching in the third week 468 mg/day (maximum dose 800 mg/day). The mean dose for imipramine was 109 mg/day in the first week and 121 mg/day in the final one (maximum dose 150 mg/day).

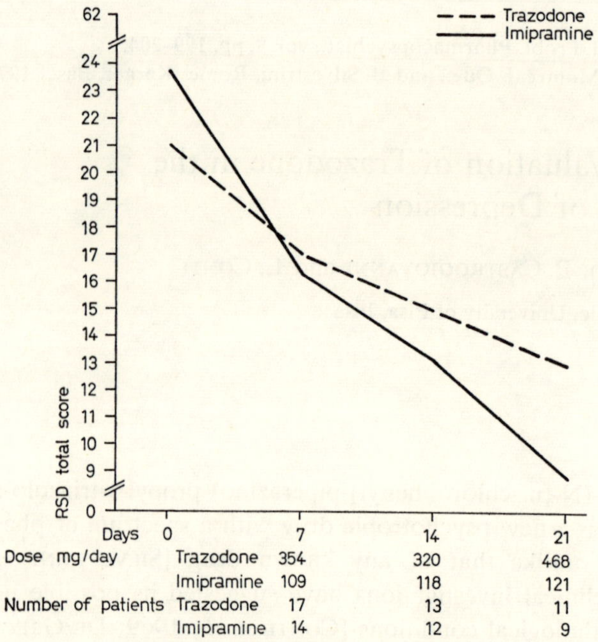

Fig. 1. The changes of the mean total scores assessed by means of the Hamilton Psychiatric Rating Scale for Depression administered to depressed inpatients during the controlled trial, are reported at different observation times.

In the pilot study changes in the symptomatology were assessed after 2, 6, 10 and 14 days of treatment by means of the Hamilton Psychiatric Rating Scale for Depression (HAM); in the controlled study after 7, 14 and 21 days by means of the HAM and the Brief Psychiatric Rating Scale (BPRS) of Overall and Gorham. The clinical judgement was expressed as 'stationary', 'worsening' or 'improvement' (slight, fair, marked) and 'recovery'.

An *all-night polygraphic recording* was performed on 6 patients in the pilot study and on 8 patients in the controlled trial.

Results and Comments

In the pilot open study 2 patients had a complete recovery, 13 improved, 2 were stationary and 3 worsened. Within the diagnostic categories the anxious depressions and the psychoneurosis had the highest rate of improvement. The mean total scores of the HAM showed significant im-

Table I. Trazodone and imipramine pre/post treatment comparison (Overall and Gorham BPRS). Discriminant and variance analysis

	Trazodone		Imipramine	
	discriminant analysis ($p = n.s.$)	variance analysis	discriminant analysis ($p = n.s.$)	variance analysis
	function	p	function	p
Anxiety	0.69	0.006	0.67	0.009
Tension	0.50	0.05	0.52	0.04
Depression	0.78	0.002	0.80	0.001

provement within two days; thus indicating a rapid activity of trazodone in spite of low doses (300 mg/day). The progressive increase of the doses did not produce a parallel rate of improvement. Similar results were obtained with several anti-anxiety benzodiazepines [CASSANO *et al.*, 1973]. The drug was found to affect mainly the anxious symptomatology 'suicide' ($p > 0.001$) and 'psychic anxiety' ($p > 0.01$) were significantly modified.

In the *controlled trial* – though according to discriminant analysis on basal scores the imipramine group was significantly more severely depressed than the other – no qualitative differences between groups were detected (variance analysis). The rapid onset of trazodone activity on anxious and depressive symptomatology previously reported [CONTI *et al.*, 1969] was confirmed (fig. 1). The mean total scores of the HAM decreased markedly both for imipramine and trazodone; patients treated with imipramine showing greater improvement. Discriminant analysis between basal and final scores of the BPRS indicated a significant improvement of 'depression', 'anxiety', and 'tension' for both compounds (table I). The HAM scores allowed a better characterization of the two drugs: trazodone acted selectively on the items 'depressive mood', 'lack of interest', 'psychic anxiety', 'somatic anxiety'; whereas imipramine showed a broader action not limited to the depressive and anxious symptomatology significantly, but also modifying 'insomnia', 'somatic gastrointestinal symptoms', 'somatic general symptoms' and 'depersonalization' (table II). Side-effects, more frequent with trazodone, did not allow a clear-cut characterization of the compound (table III). The analysis of the differences of the HAM

Table II. Trazodone and imipramine pre/post treatment comparison (Hamilton RSD). Discriminant and variance analysis

	Trazodone		Imipramine	
	discriminant analysis ($p < 0.01$)	variance analysis	discriminant analysis ($p < 0.002$)	variance analysis
	function	p	function	p
Depressive mood	0.64	0.0005	0.70	0.002
Lack of interest	0.52	0.005	0.64	0.001
Anxiety				
Psychic	0.45	0.01	0.49	0.01
Somatic	0.38	0.04	0.44	0.01
Insomnia				
Initial			0.60	0.001
Middle			0.58	0.002
Delayed			0.61	0.001
Somatic				
Gastrointestinal			0.58	0.002
General			0.50	0.008
Depersonalization			0.47	0.01

Table III. Side-effect observed during trazodone and imipramine treatment

Side-effect	Trazodone (n = 17)	Imipramine (n = 14)
Tremors	3	2
Urinary symptoms	4	–
Blurred vision	6	5
Dizziness	3	4
Headache	1	6
Dry mouth	7	2
Nausea	2	2
Constipation	2	2
Asthenia	1	1
Increased sweating	4	4
Total	36	27

Table IV. Comparison of imipramine versus trazodone, pre/post treatment score differences (Hamilton RSD). Discriminant and variance analysis

	Discriminant analysis ($p < 0.02$)	Variance analysis
	function	p
Insomnia		
Initial	0.38	0.04
Middle	0.39	0.04
Delayed	0.49	0.009
Somatic gestrointestinal	0.41	0.03

scores before and after imipramine and trazodone treatment allowed to isolate a discriminant function primarily loaded by 'insomnia' (initial, middle and delayed) and 'somatic gastrointestinal symptoms' which distinguished the two treatments (table IV). Such a result confirmed that the patients subjectively did not experience any significant improvement of insomnia during trazodone treatment. This may be explained by the EEG finding that even if the total sleep time increased, no changes in REM stage, contrary to benzodiazepines, and no increase of stage 4 as in tricyclic antidepressant treatment, were induced by trazodone. Although the controlled trial is still going on, and the present results are to be considered preliminary, consistent data were gathered to ascertain the psychotropic activity of trazodone on anxious and depressive symptomatology. The difference between imipramine and trazodone as to chemical structure and pharmacological effects on animals [SILVESTRINI *et al.*, 1969] suggest that we should set trazodone in a new class of psychoactive drugs. This is also in view of the different clinical activities. Trazodone is therefore in an intermediate position between benzodiazepines and tricyclic compounds.

References

CASSANO, G. B.; CASTROGIOVANNI, P., and CONTI, L.: Drug responses in different anxiety states under benzodiazepine treatment. Some multivariate analyses for the evaluation of 'Rating Scale for Depression' scores. The Benzodiazepine (Raven Press, New York 1973).

Conti, L.; Placidi, G. F.; Biagini, G. L., Maggini, C. e Castrogiovanni, P.: Studio clinico e poligrafico di un derivato del Triazolo 4–3-Alfa-Piridina (AF 1161). Boll. Soc. med. Chir. Pisa *3:* 226–239 (1969).

De Gregorio, M. e Dionisio, A.: Ricerche cliniche su un nuovo psicofarmaco (AF 1161). Valutazione preliminare. Med. psicosom. *14:* 477–493 (1969).

De Gregorio, M. and Dionisio, A.: A controlled clinical study of a new antidepressant (trazodone). Panminerva med. *13:* 1–2, 27–30 (1971).

Silvestrini, B.; Cioli, V.; Burberi, S., and Catanese, B.: Pharmacological properties of AF 1161, a new psychotropic drug. Int. J. Neuropharmacol. *7:* 587–599 (1968).

Authors' address: Prof. G. B. Cassano, Psychiatric Clinic, University of Pisa, *Pisa* (Italy)

Trazodone. Mod. Probl. Pharmacopsychiat., vol. 9, pp. 205–206, ed. Th. A. Ban, Montreal, Que., and B. Silvestrini, Rome (Karger, Basel 1974)

Concluding Remarks

J. SAARMA

Laboratory of Psychopharmacology, Department of Psychiatry, Tartu State University, Tartu

The First International Symposium on Trazodone has been a unique meeting. First, the entire meeting has been dealing with one single drug – trazodone. Second, the meeting has been a continuous collaboration of various specialists: biochemists, pharmacologists, toxicologists, neurophysiologists, psychologists, internists and psychiatrists. Thus, this meeting actually can be regarded as an interdisciplinary workshop on trazodone.

I think that this kind of meeting is the most fruitful way to warrant a real advancement in psychopharmacology, especially when we have to deal with a new psychotropic drug.

Excellent papers delivered at this meeting have provided us with a considerable amount of new information on trazodone, in the field of the basic sciences as well as in the field of its clinical application. Vivid discussions following the papers have contributed a great deal to the clarification of the pharmacology and clinical action of trazodone.

On the basis of data delivered at this meeting and published earlier we can conclude that trazodone is a unique psychotropic drug from many points of view.

Chemically it is quite different from all other compounds applied until now in the pharmacotherapy of psychic disorders. One can assume that trazodone may become a starting point for more triazolopyridine derivatives with psychotropic action in future.

Pharmacologically, trazodone is endowed with actions not clearly fitting into single group of drugs in the framework of generally accepted classifications. Further experiences with trazodone and with some other 'non-standard' psychotropic drugs will, obviously, contribute to revealing more appropriate pharmacological criteria for characteristics and classifications of these compounds. It is possible that this new experience and new basic data will serve as a ground for revising even our understanding of the concept and structure of depressive and anxiety states, as Dr. T. A. BAN has pointed out in his presentation.

As a psychiatrist-clinician, I am most of all concerned with the possibilities in the clinical application of trazodone. We can conclude that some significant favourable clinical features of trazodone have been established.

Trazodone has been found to be most effective in the treatment of various depressive and anxiety states. It is well known that these two forms constitute the majority among all psychic disturbances encountered in psychiatric practice, and their ratio keeps on growing. Every new effective drug can be regarded as a valuable supplement to our armoury to alleviate the suffering of these patients. In this connection, an extremely rapid onset of the therapeutic action of trazodone and its minor toxicity are especially favourable features. As we have learned at this meeting, various ways of application, e. g. intravenous infusion, can enhance markedly the favourable effects of trazodone.

There are some quite promising data on the therapeutic effect of trazodone also in some other psychic disorders, especially in patients suffering from organic brain syndrome. The importance of further studies in this direction is obvious.

Trazodone is a new drug, its pharmacological and clinical properties are far from being revealed entirely. At this meeting also a great number of questions have been asked which still are waiting for answers. I am convinced that these open questions will stimulate not only the participants of this meeting, but also numerous other colleagues to carry out further studies on trazodone.

Ladies and Gentlemen! We have spent together two fruitful days at this meeting. We owe a deep thanks to all speakers for delivering highly informative papers. We are very thankful to all colleagues who took part at discussions. Many thanks to all participants of this meeting.

These days were not only fruitful, but also very pleasant, for the meeting has been organized extremely well. I would like to express to Dr. DE SANCTIS and his staff, the deepest thanks from all of us for the excellent organization of this first International Symposium on Trazodone.

Thank you!

Author's address: Prof. J. SAARMA, MD, Chief, Laboratory of Psychopharmacology, Department of Psychiatry, Tartu State University, *Tartu, Estonian SSR* (USSR)

List of Participants and Contributors

AGNOLI, A., Department of Neurology and Psychiatry, University of Rome, Rome (Italy)

AMIN, M., Lakeshore General Hospital, Montreal (Canada)

ANGELUCCI, L., Istituto di Farmacologia e Farmacognosia, University of Rome, Piazzale delle Scienze, 5, Roma (Italy)

ANTONELLI, F., Direttore della Cattedra di Medicina Psicosomatica dell'Università Cattolica di Roma, Via della Camilluccia, 195, Roma (Italy)

BAN, T. A., Director, Division of Psychopharmacology, Department of Psychiatry, McGill University, Montreal (Canada)

BOISSIER, J. R., Unité de Neuropsychopharmacologie de l'INSERM, 2, Rue d'Alésia, F-75014 Paris (France)

CASACCHIA, M., Department of Neurology and Psychiatry, University of Rome, Rome (Italy)

CAZZULO, C., Direttore della Clinica Psichiatrica, Università di Milano, Milano (Italy)

DE GREGORIO, M., Aziende Chimiche Riunite Angelini Francesco ACRAF SpA, Viale Amelia, 70, 00181 Roma (Italy)

CASSANO, G. B., Aiuto Clinica Psichiatrica dell'Università di Pisa, Pisa (Italy)

DIONISIO, A., Aziende Chimiche Riunite Angelini Francesco ACRAF SpA, Viale Amelia, 70, 00181 Roma (Italy)

DOMINO, E. F., Department of Pharmacology, University of Michigan, Ann Arbor (USA)

FAZIO, C., Direttore, 1A Clinica Delle Malattie Nervose e Mentali Della Università di Roma, Viale dell'Università 30, Roma (Italy)

FUJITA, T., Head Biochemistry Department, Eisai Co. Ltd., Tokyo (Japan)

GALVAN, L., Director, Experimental Psychopharmacological Unit, Instituto Nacional de Neurologia, Mexico City, Mexico D. F. (Mexico)

GARATTINI, S., Direttore, Istituto di Recerche Farmacologiche «Mario Negri», Via Eritrea, 62, Milano (Italy)

GATTI, G., Primo Ricercatore, Istituto Superiore di Sanità, Viale Regina Elena, 299, Roma (Italy)

GUNELLA, G., Primario, Servizio di Fisiopatologia Respiratoria e Terapia Medica dell'Insufficienza Respiratorio Cronica, Policlinico S. Orsola, University of Bologna, Bologna (Italy)

HAJDU, A., Montreal Children's Hospital, Montreal (Canada)

LAPIERRE, Y., Scientific Director, Hôpital Pierre Janet, Hull (Canada)

LING, G., Professor and Head, Department of Pharmacology, The Faculty of Medicine, University of Ottawa, Ottawa (Canada)

LONGO, V. G., Istituto Superiore di Sanità, Viale Regina Elena 299, 00181 Roma (Italy)

LOPEZ ZANON, A., Director de la Clínica Psiquiátrica de la Policlínica Francisco Franco de Madrid, Madrid (Spain)

MIURA, S., Associate Professor of Psychiatry Medical School, Kitazato University, Sagamihara (Japan)

MONTANINI, R., Primario, Neurologo dell'Ospedale Civ. S. Antonio Abate, Gallarate, Milano (Italy)

MURATORIO, A., Direttore dell'Ospedale Psichiatrico dell'Aquila e Professore incaricato della Clinica Psichiatrica dell'Università di Pisa, Pisa (Italy)

NAIR, N. P. V., Douglas Hospital, Montreal (Canada)

PARIANTE, F., Direttore dell'Ospedale Psichiatrico di Volterra, Pisa (Italy)

PERUZY, D., Incaricato di Statistica Sanitaria dell'Università di Roma, c/o Ospedale Forlanini, Roma (Italy)

PICCIONE, M., Department of Neurology and Psychiatry, University of Rome, Rome (Italy)

RADUCO-THOMAS, C., Chairman and Professor, Department of Psychopharmacology, Laval University, Quebec City (Canada)

RINALDI, F., Direttore, Clinica Malattie Nervose e Mentali di Bari, Bari (Italy)

RIVETT, K. F., Deputy Director of Toxicology, Huntingdon Research Center, Huntingdon (England)

SAARMA, J., Chairman, Department of Psychiatry, Tartu State University, Estonian S.S.R. (USSR)

SCHWARZ, DIETER, Max-Planck-Institut für Psychiatrie, Hamburg (West Germany)

SCORZA-BARCELLONA, P., Aziende Chimiche Riunite Angelini Francesco ACRAF SpA, Viale Amelia, 70, 00181 Roma (Italy)

SHIBAHARA, T., Director, Department of Psychiatry, Kyoto First Red Cross Hospital, Kyoto (Japan)

SILVESTRINI, B., Aziende Chimiche Riunite Angelini Francesco ACRAF SpA, Viale Amelia, 70, 00181 Roma (Italy)

ST. LAURENT, J., Associate Professor, Department of Psychiatry, Université de Sherbrooke, Sherbrooke (Canada)

SUZUKI, Y., Toxicologist, Eisai Co. Ltd., Tokyo (Japan)

VERGARA, L. E., Director Médico, Hospital Psiquiátrico Nacional, Panama (Rep. de Panama)

VILLENEUVE, A., Chief, Research Department, Hôpital Saint Michel Archange, Quebec City (Canada)

WHEATLEY, D. P. (Middlesex/England)

YAMATSU, K., Pharmacologist, Eisai Co. Ltd., Tokyo (Japan)

Subject Index